kama
sutra
365

kama
sutra
365

London, New York, Melbourne, Munich, Delhi

Editor: Katey Mackenzie
Designer: Alison Fenton
Project Editor: Daniel Mills
Project Art Editor: Natasha Montgomery
Executive Managing Editor: Adèle Hayward
Managing Art Editor: Kat Mead
Production Editor: Jenny Woodcock
Production Controller: Mandy Inness
Creative Technical Support: Sonia Charbonnier
Art Director: Peter Luff
Publisher: Stephanie Jackson

First American Edition, 2008

Published in the United States by
DK Publishing
375 Hudson Street
New York, New York 10014

08 09 10 11   10 9 8 7 6 5 4 3 2 1

KD126—November 2008

Published in Great Britain by Dorling Kindersley Limited.
A catalog record for this book is available from the Library of Congress.
ISBN 978-0-7566-3979-2

DK books are available at special discounts when purchased in bulk for sales promotions, premiums, fund-
raising, or educational use. For details, contact: DK Publishing Special Markets, 375 Hudson Street, New York,
New York 10014 or SpecialSales@dk.com.

Color reproduction by Colourscan, Singapore, and MDP, Bath, UK
Printed and bound in Singapore by Star Standard

PUBLISHER'S NOTE: Neither the publisher nor the author is engaged in rendering professional advice or
services to the individual reader, and neither shall be liable or responsible for any loss or damage allegedly
arising from any information or suggestion in this book. All participants in such activities must assume the
responsibility for their own actions and safety and for compliance with all applicable laws. If you have any
health problems or medical conditions or any other concerns about whether you are able to participate in
any of these activities, you should take appropriate precautions. The information contained in this book
cannot replace professional advice or sound judgment and good decision making, nor does the scope of
this book allow for disclosure of all the potential hazards and risks involved in such activities.

Discover more at www.dk.com

Contents

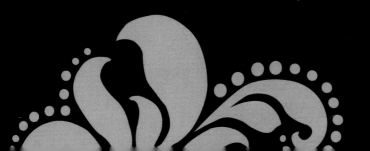

Introduction

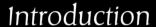

Welcome to Kama Sutra 365—the book that celebrates
Eastern sex positions in all their naughty, up-against-the-
wall, down-on-all-fours glory, including classic exotic
suggestions for warming up before, and for cooling down
after. Whether you're bringing home a hot new date or
putting the passion back into a decades-old marriage,
there's a position for you. And, with 365 positions, you can
go for a whole glorious year without repeating yourself—
or, if you have sex once a week, for seven years.

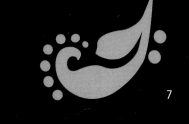

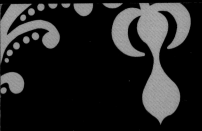

The Kama Sutra

The Kama Sutra was written in ancient India by Vatsyayana Malanaga. He reveals not only the best positions in which to have sex, but also how to embrace, kiss, and even bite. He describes how a room should be prepared for lovemaking and the etiquette two lovers should employ.

Kama Sutra sex tip: "Put his whole lingam (penis) into your mouth and press it to the very end as if you are going to swallow it."

The Ananga Ranga

This was written in 15th-century India by Kalyana Malla. Unlike the Kama Sutra, which was intended for all lovers, the Ananga Ranga speaks directly to husbands and wives. Its core message is to keep sex varied and adventurous so that husband and wife aren't tempted to stray into "polygamy, adultery, and every other manner of vice."

Ananga Ranga sex tip: "To perfect her husband's pleasure, a wife should constrict her yoni (vagina) so it holds the lingam (penis) tight."

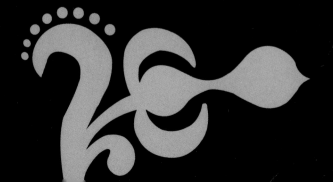

The Perfumed Garden

Written by Sheikh Nefzawi in 16th-century Tunis, this Arabic love manual tells lovers not just how to make love—and in what position—but also what desirable features to seek in the genitals of the opposite sex.

Perfumed Garden sex tip: "The 'quencher' is the penis that fully satisfies a woman's amorous desires because it is thick and strong, and slow to ejaculate."

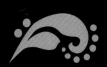

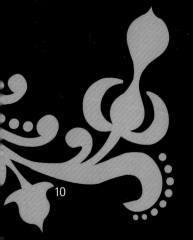

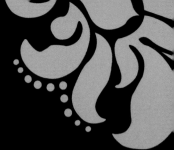

The Tao

This is a collection of Taoist writings from ancient China. The Taoist view of sex is that it's essential for good health, bringing mental, physical, and even spiritual well-being. This is because when you have sex, your yin (female energy) and yang (male energy) become harmonized.

Tao sex tip: "Slowly insert your penis five inches into her vagina and then slowly withdraw."

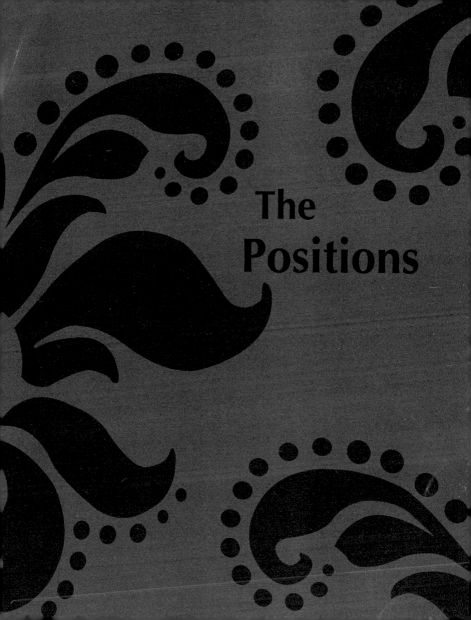

The
Positions

The shampooer

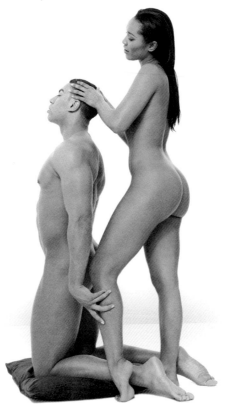

She massages his scalp in gentle shampooing movements.

Divine moment: Make the most of having him at your fingertips.
Pure nirvana: Rub fragrant coconut oil into his scalp.

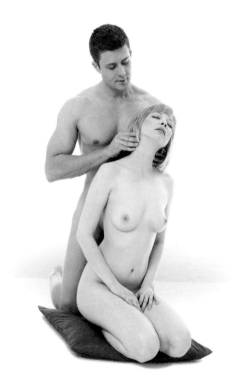

He presses his fingertips into the muscles at the sides of her neck.

Divine moment: Add your lips to the equation.
Pure nirvana: Run your fingers through her hair
and hold her head in your hands.

3   Embrace of the calf

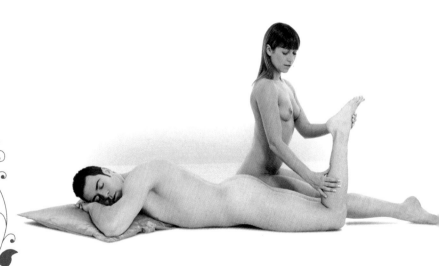

She smoothes her thumb along the length of his calf muscle.

Divine moment: Plant soulful kisses on the bottom of his foot.
Pure nirvana: Take your fingers on a cheeky walk to his butt.

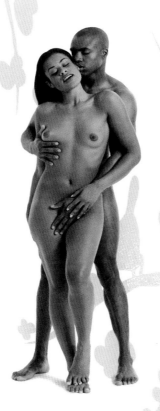

He approaches from behind, wraps his arms around her, and caresses her breast.

Divine moment: Exploit the take-her-by-surprise factor—
sidle up when she's not expecting it.
Pure nirvana: Guide his hand to your bliss button.

5 The awakener

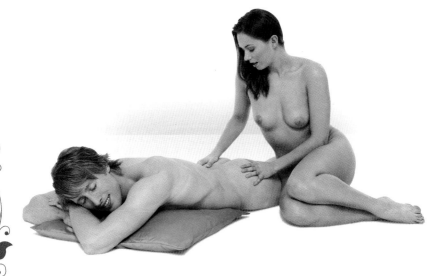

She takes his buttocks firmly in hand as she presses,
strokes, scratches, and kneads.

Divine moment: Add some sexy buttock nibbles to your wake-up call.
Pure nirvana: Lean forward—use your breasts like another pair of hands.

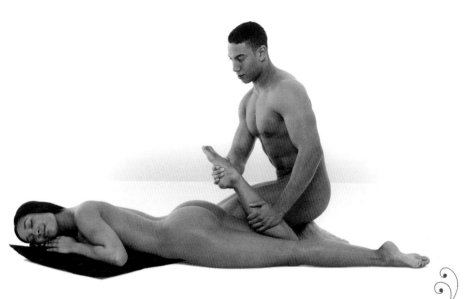

He massages her feet with warm oil as she lies on her belly.

Divine moment: Say, "Trust me, I'm a reflexologist."
Pure nirvana: Press her "sex reflex"—the bony part
under the inside of her ankle.

7 The lion tamer

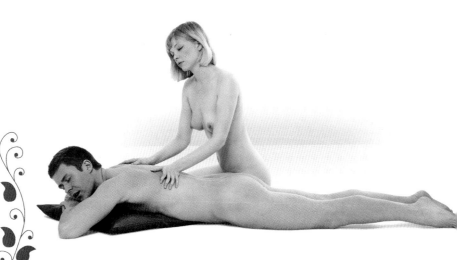

She presses and rubs her palms along the length of his back as he lies forward.

Divine moment: Drip warm oil between his shoulder blades, and
let it trickle down the length of his spine.
Pure nirvana: Roll him over at the end to charm his snake.

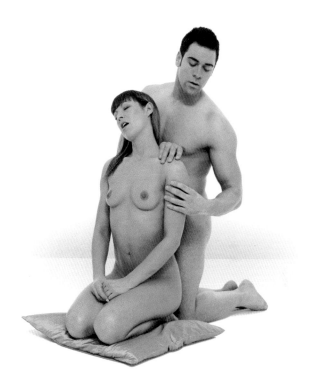

He kneels behind her to deliver a firm but sensual shoulder rub.

Divine moment: Say, "Mmmm, darling, I could do this all night."
Pure nirvana: Feed her chocolate-covered strawberries at the same time.

Prowling tigress

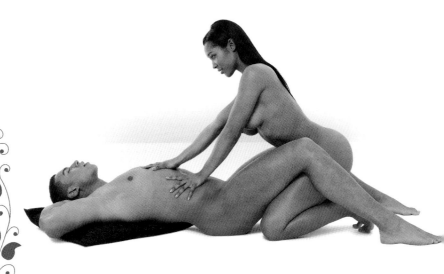

*She kneels between his legs, leans in toward him
and slides her hands along his belly and chest.*

Divine moment: Do your best predatory cat impression.
Pure nirvana: Claw and rake his chest.

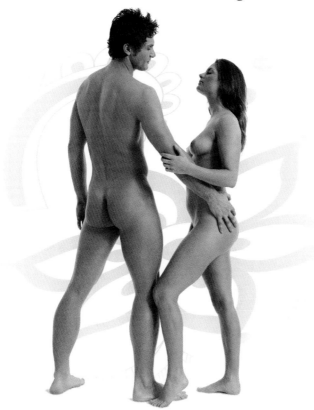

He finds some pretext to move in close and touch her body.

Divine moment: Make your approach warm and friendly.
Pure nirvana: Yet have a saucy twinkle in your eye....

11   The rubbing embrace

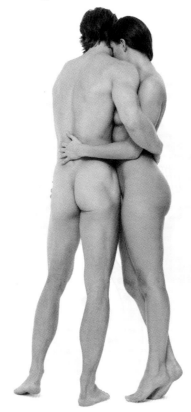

They slip off in a dark or crowded place, and grind against each other.

Divine moment: Say, "Do you want to come up for coffee?"
Pure nirvana: Make out like teenagers.

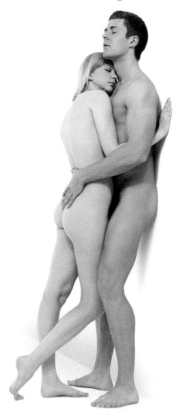

She pins his body against a wall or a pillar, and pushes herself against him.

Divine moment: Press your bits hard against his hard bits.
Pure nirvana: Suggest trying the horizontal version.

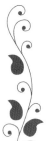

13 The piercing embrace

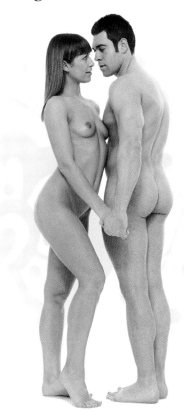

She presses her breasts against him "as if trying to pierce him with her nipples."

Divine moment: Ask him what he's doing later.
Pure nirvana: Tease him by pulling away.

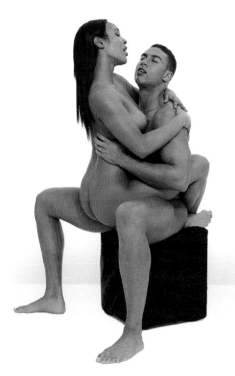

Blind with passion, they embrace each other as if they "want to enter each other's body." (Only for couples who are "already moist.")

Divine moment: He grabs her ass, and pulls her even closer.
Pure nirvana: Oops—his lingam slips into her yoni.

Mixture of rice and sesame

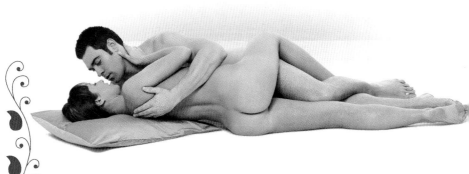

They lie down in a tight embrace, bodies as closely intertwined as a mixture of rice and sesame.

Divine moment: Do it with someone you've just met at a party.
Pure nirvana: Frot shamelessly.

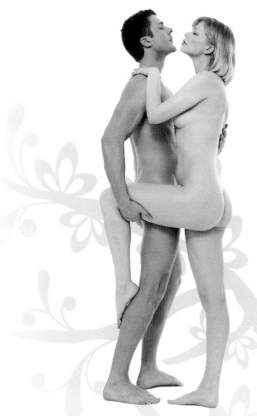

*She presses her foot against the back of his leg
as if climbing his body with desire.*

Divine moment: Ask if he's got a firm branch you can sit on.
Pure nirvana: Pick her up, and carry her to bed.

Twining of the creeper

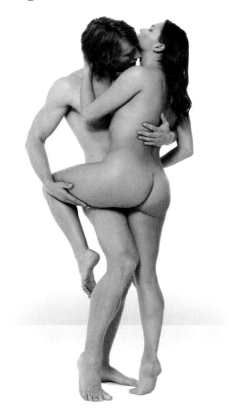

She winds herself around him "like a vine twines around the great dammar tree."

Divine moment: Cling tightly to one other.
Pure nirvana: Bask in the knowledge that sex is a sure thing.

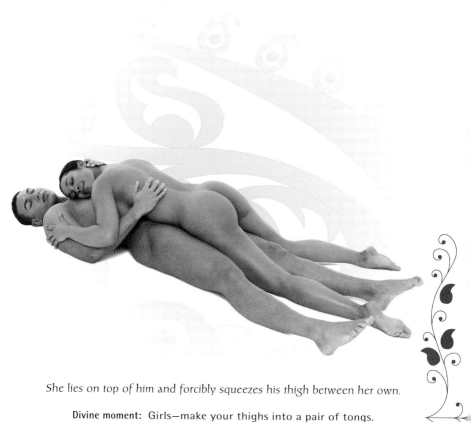

She lies on top of him and forcibly squeezes his thigh between her own.

Divine moment: Girls—make your thighs into a pair of tongs.
Pure nirvana: Bend your knee to get a tight thigh-to-genital fit.

19 Embrace of the jaghana

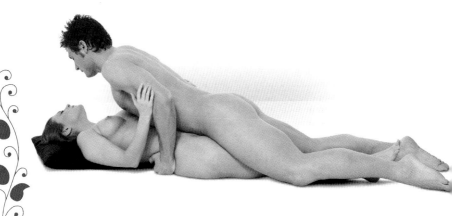

He climbs on top and presses the middle part (jaghana)
of her body with his own.

Divine moment: Savor those pre-penetration sensations.
Pure nirvana: Look into her eyes as you make your entrance.

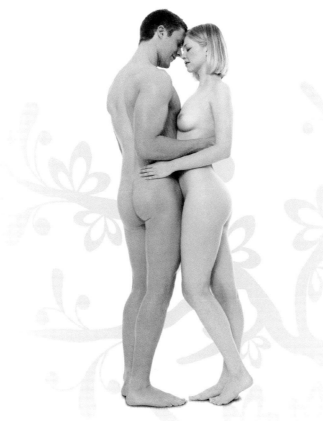

They lean toward each other, eyes closed and foreheads touching.

Divine moment: Tune in to your third-eye chakras.
Pure nirvana: Talk dirty by telepathy.

21 Embrace of the breasts

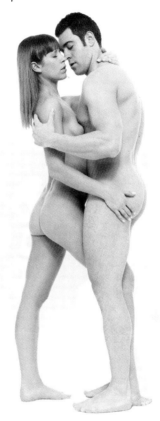

They stand face to face and press their chests against each other.

Divine moment: Do it while dancing to Barry White.
Pure nirvana: Move your hips in sync.

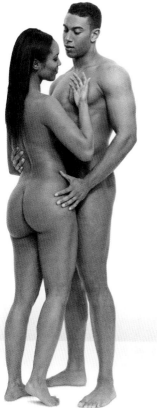

She uses the back of her hand to slap him playfully on the chest.

Divine moment: Tell him what a *very* naughty boy he's been.
Pure nirvana: Up the kink-factor by wearing a bondage-style outfit.

23   *Striking with the fingers contracted*

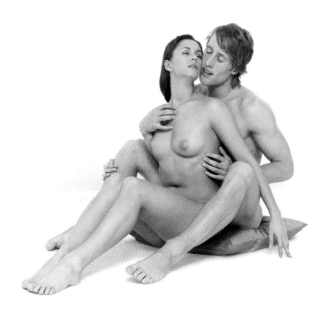

He raps her lightly between her breasts with his fingers slightly bent.

Divine moment: Make it sensual not sadistic.
Pure nirvana: Patter your fingertips like raindrops across her skin.

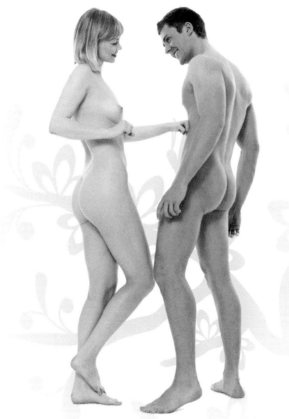

She delivers a playful punch in the abs.

Divine moment: Tell her how hot she is when she's angry.
Pure nirvana: Suggest you resolve this in the bedroom.

25 Open-hand strike

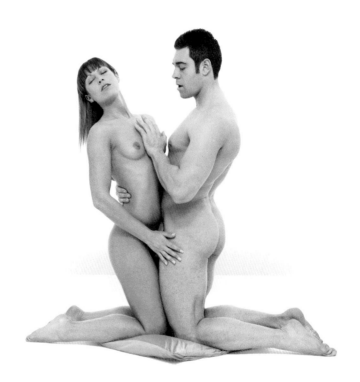

He lightly slaps her with his palm (note: it's gentlemanly to ask first).

Divine moment: Turn her round so her bum's in the air—*now* get spanky.
Pure nirvana: Follow each butt-spank with a friendly massage.

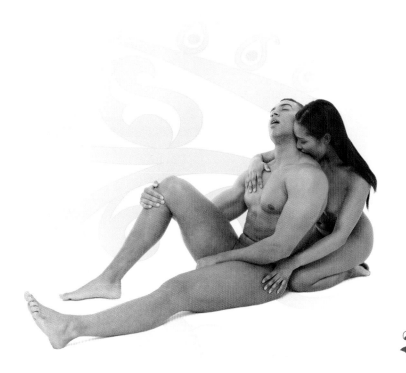

She bites him repeatedly on the shoulder or chest, leaving a row of red marks.

Divine moment: Do it at the height of passion (the *Kama Sutra* says
this is "only for couples whose sexual energy is fierce").
Pure nirvana: If he's a pain junkie, dig your nails into his chest too.

The broken cloud

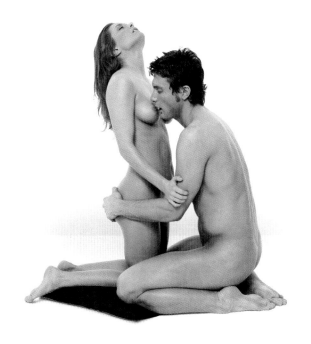

He gently nibbles her breast to create a circular mark.

Divine moment: ...Or make your mark by sucking.
Pure nirvana: Take your tongue on a detour to her nipple.

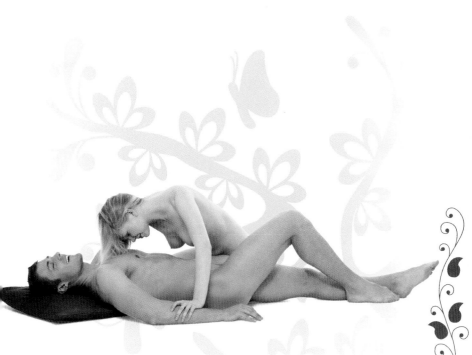

She wafts her hair sensuously over his chest and belly.

Divine moment: Let your nipples graze his skin too.
Pure nirvana: Coil your hair around his erect penis, and then pull away.

29 The polished earring

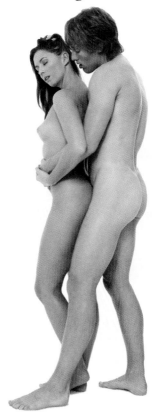

He lifts her hair to find the erogenous zone along the back of her ear and neck.

Divine moment: Caress her neck with hot, slow (fragrant) breath.
Pure nirvana: Take her earlobe between your lips, and trace the outline with your tongue.

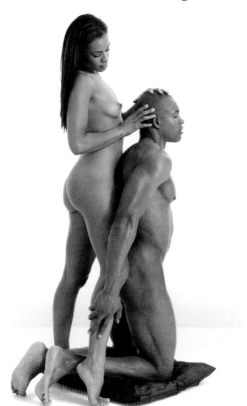

She gently runs her fingertips through his hair or over the contours of his scalp.

Divine moment: Casually lean your thigh and pelvis into his back.
Pure nirvana: Stroke his earlobes and jawline.

The bent kiss

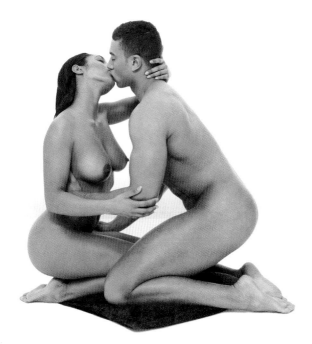

They bend their heads so they can get close, and kiss passionately.

Divine moment: Get lost in kissing—"moderation will not be necessary".
Pure nirvana: Gently tug on each other's hair as you reach
a passionate crescendo.

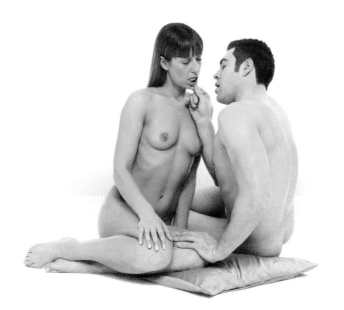

He presses her lower lip between finger and thumb before moving in to kiss her.

Divine moment: Wet your fingertip in her mouth
then trace the outline of her lips.
Pure nirvana: Do some light lip-sucking.

33 The straight kiss

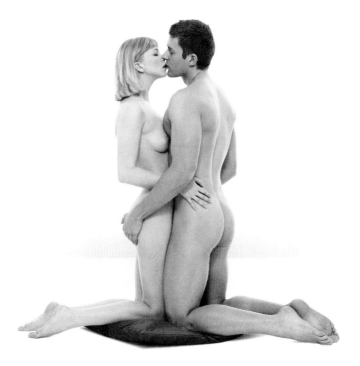

Their faces touch, and their partly opened lips meet.

Divine moment: Don't play tonsil hockey—savor the lip-on-lip feeling.
Pure nirvana: Whisper into her mouth.

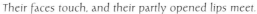

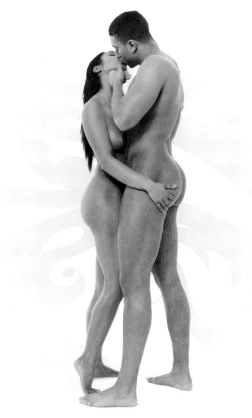

He raises her chin with his hand to kiss her mouth.

Divine moment: Softly pinch her earlobe as you kiss.
Pure nirvana: Give him a good buttock grope.

The kiss of the upper lip

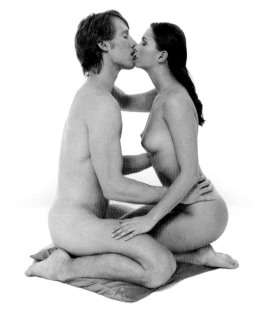

He kisses her upper lip as she kisses his lower lip.

Divine moment: Nibble his lower lip like it's an earlobe.
Pure nirvana: Ramp up the romance—cup her face in your hands.

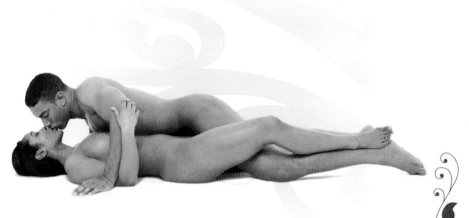

She encloses both of his lips in both of hers.
("Avoid if he has a mustache" says the Kama Sutra.)

Divine moment: Tease him with brief flicks of your tongue.
Pure nirvana: As the kiss heats up, gently suck his tongue into your mouth.

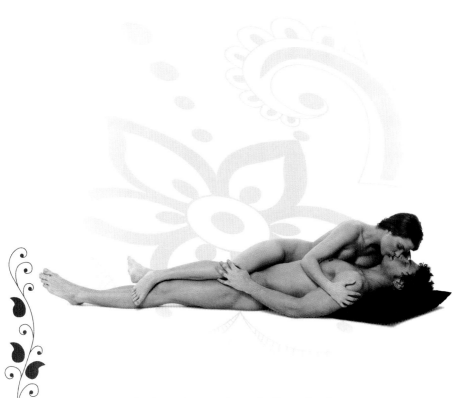

She kisses him gently on the lips as he sleeps.

Divine moment: Take your kisses southbound.
Pure nirvana: To truly kindle love, pop him in your mouth as he awakes.

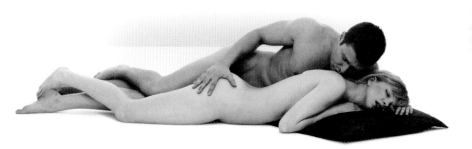

He comes home, full of desire, and wakes her with soft kisses.

Divine moment: Moan encouragingly, but make him wait before you respond.
Pure nirvana: When you're ready to receive a guest, turn over sleepily....

The kiss that turns away

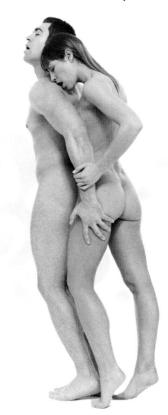

She kisses him when he's turned away from her. Her aim: to get his attention.

Divine moment: Seduce his body with nuzzling and stroking.
Pure nirvana: Seduce his mind with an indecent proposal.

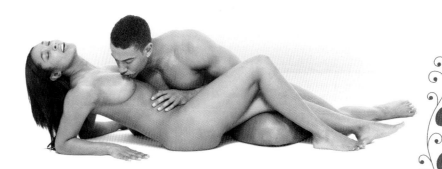

He sprinkles her breasts with seductive kisses in the build-up to sex.

Divine moment: Make her nipple the pinnacle of your act.
Pure nirvana: Share the love—mouth on one breast, fingers on the other.

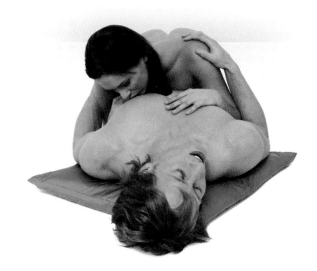

She lies on top of him, and drops feather-light kisses on his skin.

Divine moment: Lick his skin, and then blow on it.
Pure nirvana: Kiss and lick the insides of his thighs.

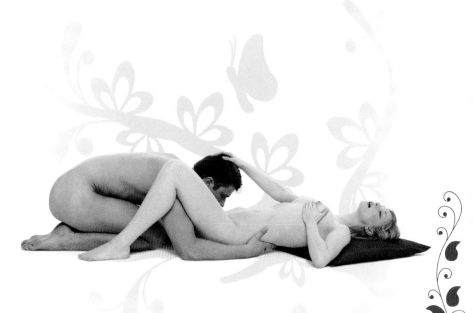

He kneels between her legs, and swirls his tongue on her terrace.

Divine moment: Once you've found her jewel,
shake your head from side to side.
Pure nirvana: Getting oral fatigue? Wear a tongue vibrator.

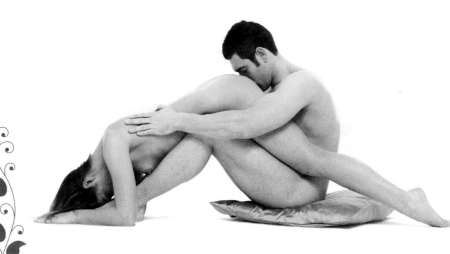

She drapes herself over his knees, and he applies his tongue to her yoni.

Divine moment: Guys—go for full immersion.
Pure nirvana: Visit all three beauty spots—clitoris, vagina, and anus.

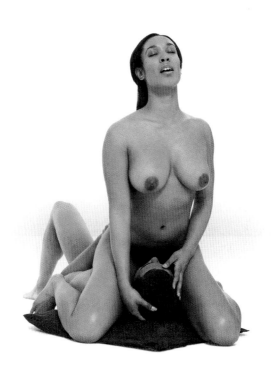

Shakti adopts a kneeling position over Shiva's face.

Divine moment: Shaktis—lean forward and take the weight on your hands.
Pure nirvana: Shivas—suck, lick, flick, and swirl to deliver a sacred orgasm.

Drinking from the source

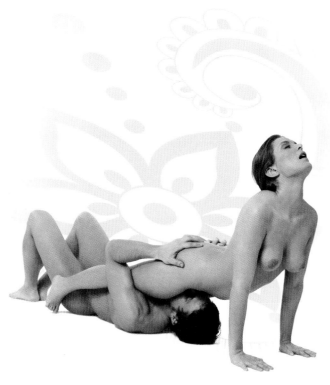

She does a push-up over his face while he sips from the source.

Divine moment: It's a quickie—turn your tongue to
maximum speed setting.
Pure nirvana: Get your whole face in on the act.

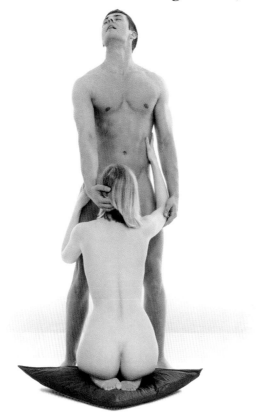

He stands. She kneels. She takes him in her mouth.

Divine moment: Surprise him by doing it in the shower.
Pure nirvana: Use your mouth and hands together to polish his pillar.

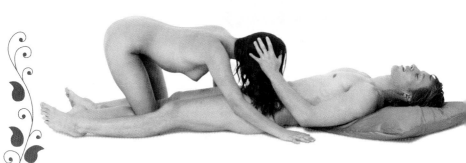

She gets on all fours, and uses her mouth to make his snake rise.

Divine moment: Slap him against your cheek, porn style.
Pure nirvana: Hold a mini-vibrator against his balls.

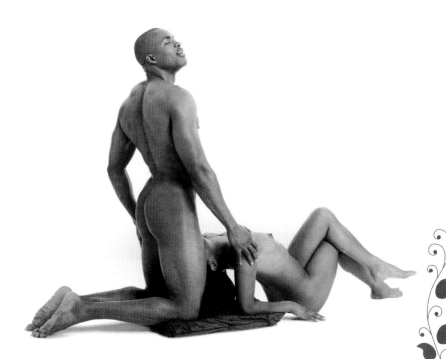

She sits in front of him, and backbends her way to a blow job.

Divine moment: Now's the time for tongue yoga.
Pure nirvana: If you've mastered your gag reflex, follow with deep throat.

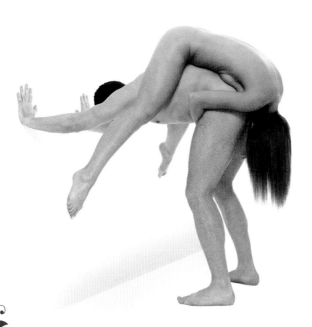

She straddles his back, and takes the back-door approach to oral sex.

Divine moment: Guys—bend your head to catch the view.
Pure nirvana: If his jade stem won't stretch, try analingus instead.

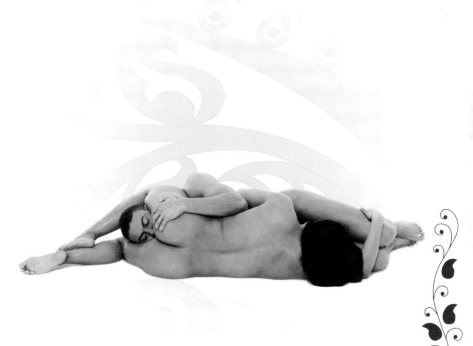

They pay each other lip service by lying on their sides,
heads aligned with each other's genitals.

Divine moment: Get into a joint rhythm, and work up a head-banging pace.
Pure nirvana: Try the foot fetishist's version—tongues to toes.

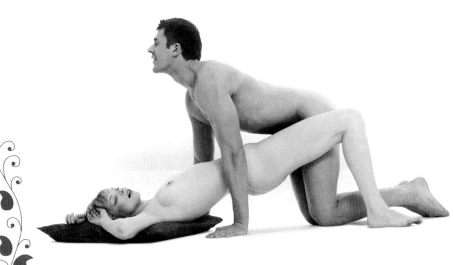

*She raises her hips high in the air, and he gets on all fours
between her open legs.*

Divine moment: Place a gentlemanly hand in the small of her back.
Pure nirvana: Instruct him to stay still while you rise and fall on his member.

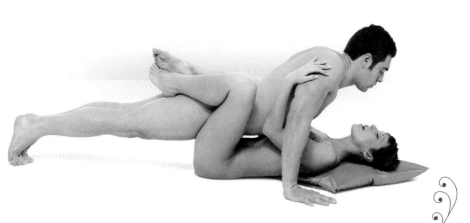

He enters her in a push-up position, and she wraps her legs around his body.

Divine moment: Guys—treat it as a workout: minimum 100 push-ups.
Pure nirvana: Pull him in tight with your legs when he comes.

53   Fish in the river

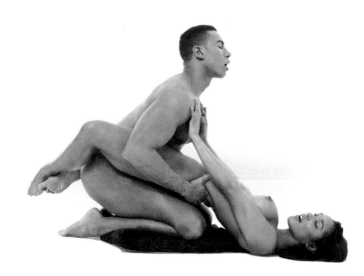

He kneels on a cushion. She sits astride him, clasps his shoulders,
and leans back until her head touches the floor.

Divine moment: Girls—try some fish-like undulations.
Pure nirvana: Enjoy the rush of blood to the head.

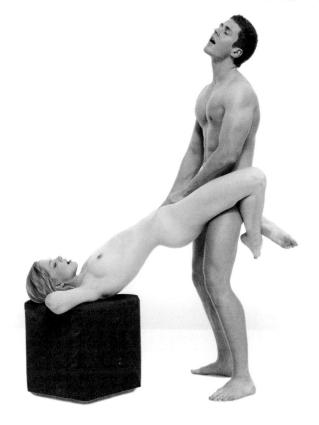

*She rests her head and shoulders on the edge of the bed
as he stands and penetrates.*

Divine moment: Use a sex sling to make it viable.
Pure nirvana: Help her down, and give her a hand-delivered orgasm.

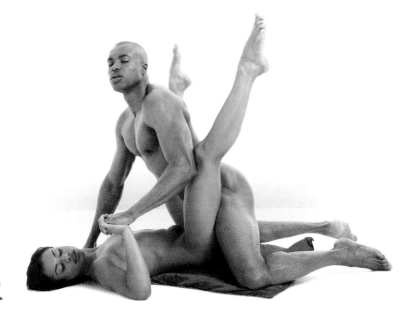

She lies on her back, and parts her legs in the widest "V" she can manage.

Divine moment: Prepare for deeeeeep penetration.
Pure nirvana: It's high on porn-chic—videotape yourselves.

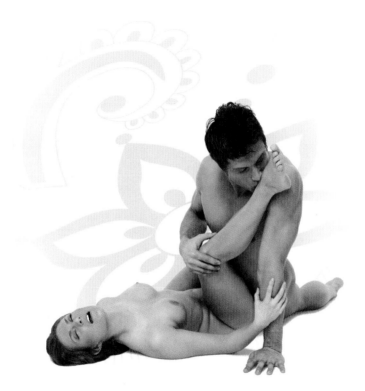

She rests one foot on his shoulder as he enters her.

Divine moment: Plant a row of kisses along her silky calf.
Pure nirvana: Girls—make sure your legs are at their buffed best.

57 Piercing the fruit

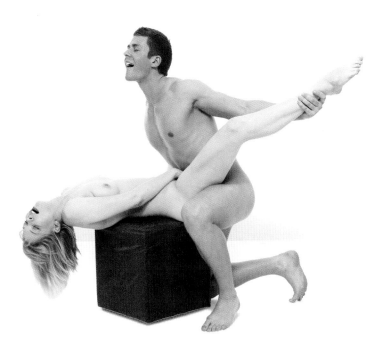

He half-kneels/half-squats, and presses himself between her widely parted legs.

Divine moment: He comes over all dominant.
Pure nirvana: She drops her legs if she gets groin strain.

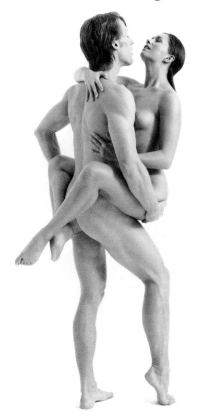

She wraps her legs around his waist, and hugs his top half.

Divine moment: He adopts a pose of mountain-like stability.
Pure nirvana: Impress with your ability to carry her *and* thrust.

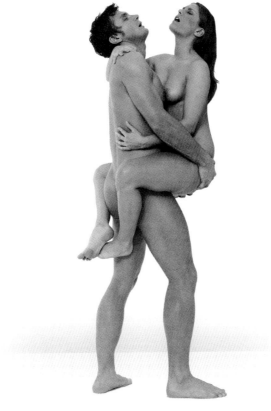

*He carries her in his arms, and presses her back against a wall,
pillar, column, or tree.*

Divine moment: Make it the follow-up to Ascending the Mountain (no. 58).
Pure nirvana: Girls—let *his* pillar take some of your weight too.

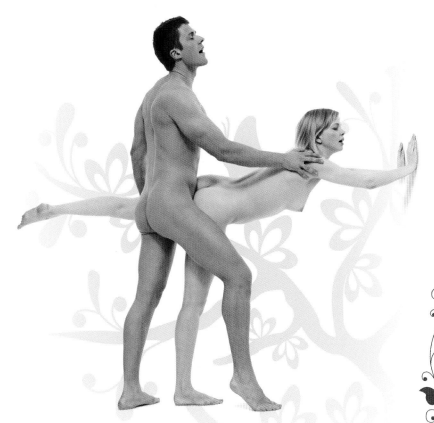

She presses her hands against a wall, and stretches her leg out behind her as he penetrates in a standing position.

Divine moment: He supports her raised thigh...
Pure nirvana: ...and fires her from his taut bow.

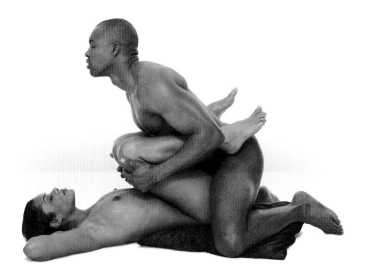

She lies back, and rests her heels on his ass while he kneels.

Divine moment: Push her knees together to get a snug fit.
Pure nirvana: Make it your raunchy opening move on a one-night stand.

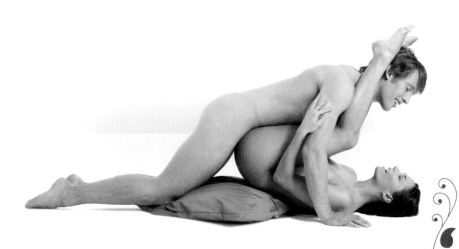

She brings her knees to her chest, and raises her ass in the air; he lies on top.

Divine moment: Start in missionary, and gradually move your legs higher.
Pure nirvana: Feel smug about being so supple.

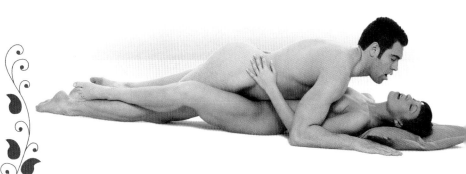

He goes on top, and she hooks her heels around his calves.

Divine moment: Move your manhood like a piston against her clitoris.
Pure nirvana: Get in a groove, and don't stop.

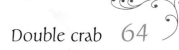

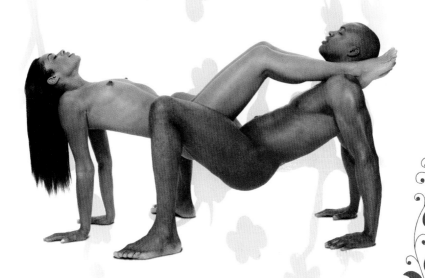

He supports himself in a crab position while she puts her feet on his shoulders.

Divine moment: Do it in front of an audience.
Pure nirvana: Don't bother keeping a straight face.

Lotus-like position

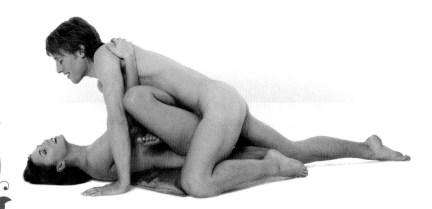

She gets into the lotus position while lying down—he climbs on top.

Divine moment: Do it with your yoga instructor after class.
Pure nirvana: Chant "*om*" as you reach orgasm.

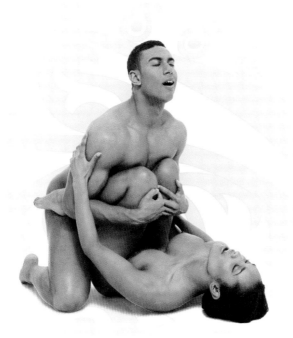

She lies down, and draws her knees up to her body.
He presses himself forward on her legs.

Divine moment: Enjoy the sensation of being near yet far.
Pure nirvana: Unwind in this position after a hard day at the office.

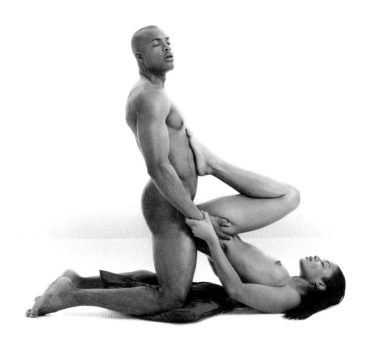

*She presses the soles of her feet on his front
and he lifts her onto his manhood.*

Divine moment: Tell Indra how hot he looks.
Pure nirvana: Wives—show off by putting your feet behind your head.

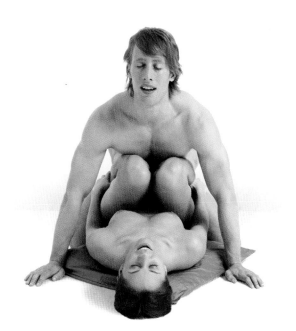

He enters on top as she clasps her ankles and pulls them near her ass.

Divine moment: Say "I've got you covered, darling."
Pure nirvana: Girls—squeeze him from the inside.

Half-pressed position

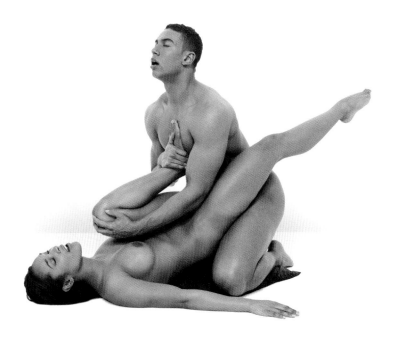

She lies between his legs, puts one foot on his chest,
and points the other leg out behind him.

Divine moment: Girls—if you like toe nibbling, slide your foot higher.
Pure nirvana: Guys—mix up your strokes. Shallow for five, then deep for five.

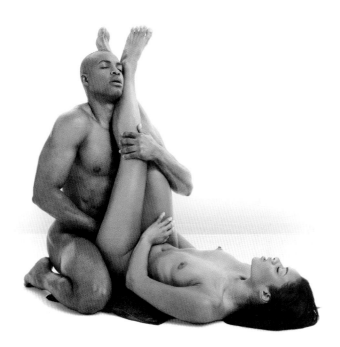

*She lies back with her legs over one of his shoulders
and her ass nestled tightly between his legs.*

Divine moment: Now she's put her feet up, tell her an erotic bedtime story.
Pure nirvana: Put your hand to good use between her legs.

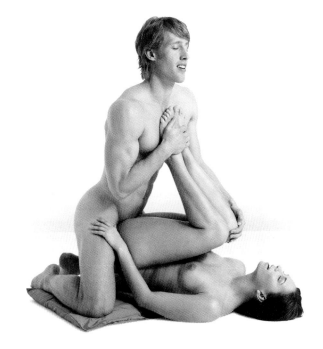

She lies on her back with her feet pressed against his chest as he bears forward.

Divine moment: Slide in deliciously slowly.
Pure nirvana: Rub your hands up and down his thighs.

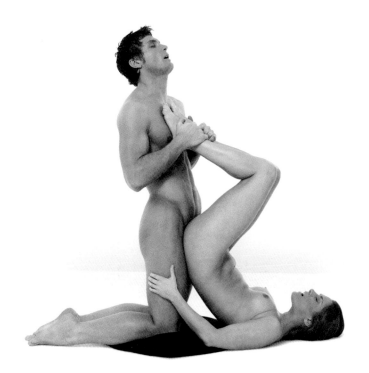

He enters her as she does a half-shoulderstand—her feet rest on his chest.

Divine moment: Say, "Let's make beautiful music."
Pure nirvana: Girls—bring your knees closer to your head
to get him in deeper.

73   Splitting the bamboo

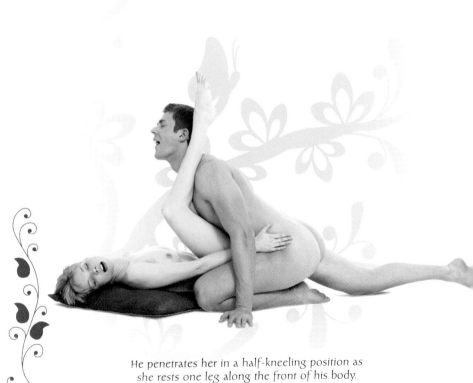

*He penetrates her in a half-kneeling position as
she rests one leg along the front of his body.*

Divine moment: Drop your inhibitions—moan/scream/shout.
Pure nirvana: Surprise him with a mid-sex spank.

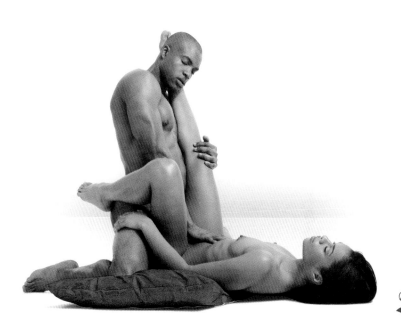

She points one foot toward the ceiling, and rests the other on his bum
as he enters her in a kneeling position.

Divine moment: Take control—manipulate her legs into position.
Pure nirvana: Use your hand to show how cliterate you are.

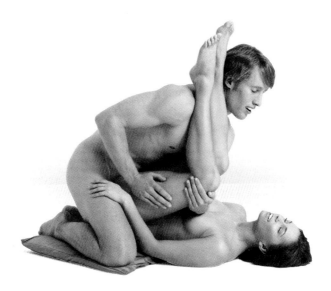

She brings her knees to her chest, and rests her calves on
one of his shoulders as he bears down on top of her.

Divine moment: Compact sex at its best—do it in a tent.
Pure nirvana: Crawl out, and lie under the stars together.

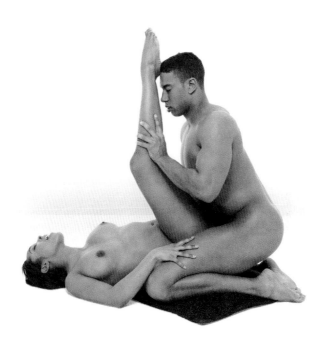

She pushes her heel (the hammer) against his head (the nail) as he enters her in a kneeling position.

Divine moment: Ladies—relish the lying-down dominance.
Pure nirvana: Gents—shout when your nail's coming through the wall.

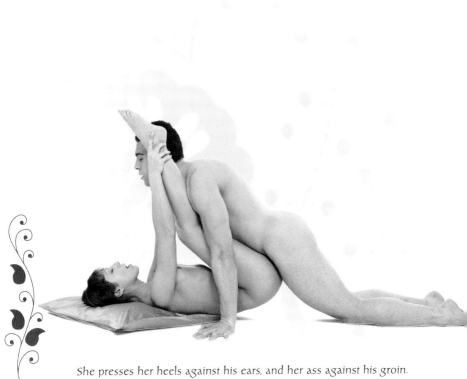

She presses her heels against his ears, and her ass against his groin.

Divine moment: Guys—take a few shallow dips before you go in deep.
Pure nirvana: Once you're in, move with abandon.

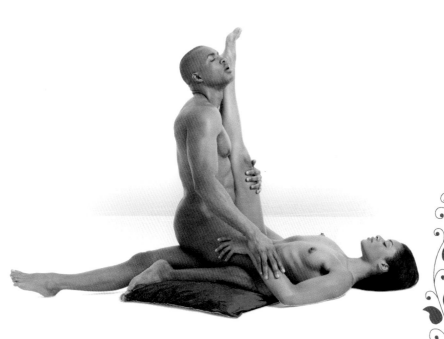

She puts one leg in the air and one flat on the bed as he penetrates.

Divine moment: Kink things up with a pair of stockings and heels.
Pure nirvana: Peel back the stocking, and give her a post-coital leg massage.

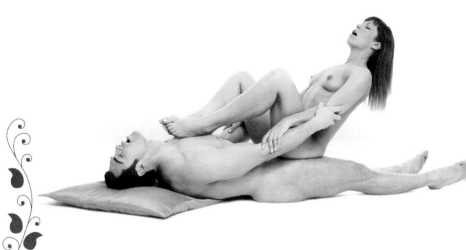

She sits on his prone body with the soles of her feet pressed together.

Divine moment: Up the challenge by doing it on a water bed.
Pure nirvana: Managed more than 20 seconds? Reward yourself.

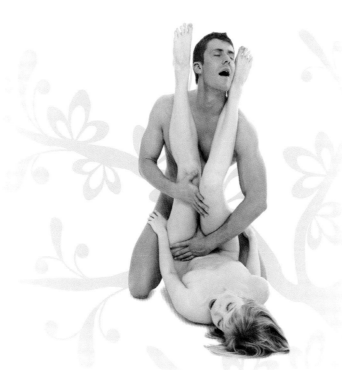

He kneels upright, and she props her legs against him in a tight "V" shape.

Divine moment: He does some clever handiwork with his thumb.
Pure nirvana: Raise the game with pillows under her butt.

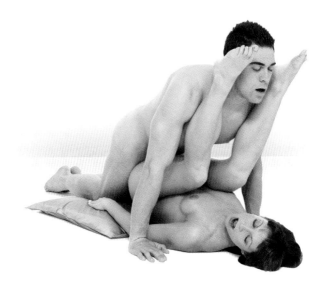

She embraces his head with her feet as he kneels over her.

Divine moment: Girls—do it when you want to maximize his length.
Pure nirvana: Touch your nipples with your knees.

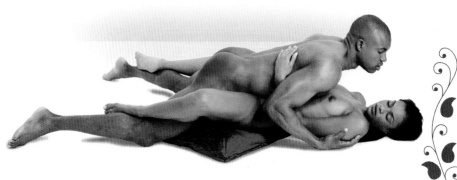

She hooks her legs over his in the missionary position.

Divine moment: Ride high on her body for best penis–clitoris contact.
Pure nirvana: Girls—get him to almost withdraw. Now circle your pelvis.

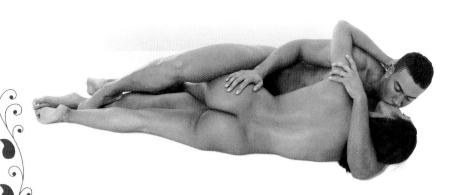

They lie holding each other—her upper thigh between both of his.

Divine moment: Do it under a blanket on a quiet bit of beach.
Pure nirvana: Keep your moves small and subtle.

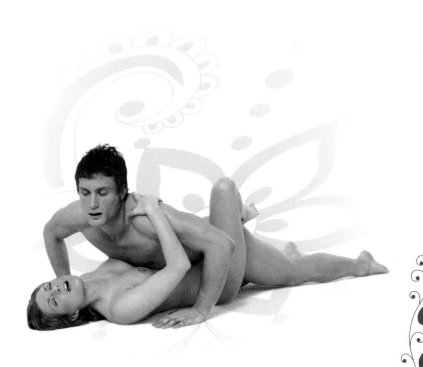

She twines her arms and legs around his body as he lies on top.

Divine moment: Make this your climax scene.
Pure nirvana: Girls—use your heel to have a say in the pace.

85 Goat on a mountain path

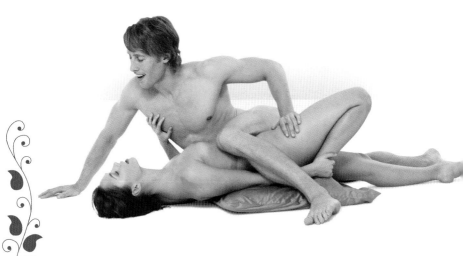

She holds her ankle against her ass while he scales her body from the side.

Divine moment: Cooperate to get to the peak.
Pure nirvana: Revert to missionary if the going gets tough.

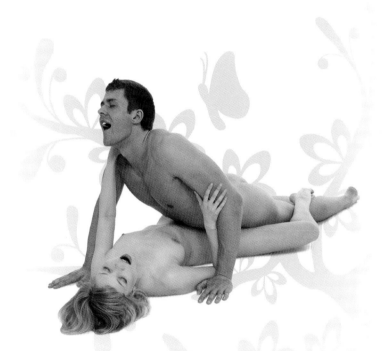

She hooks her leg over the back of his as he penetrates in a push-up position.

Divine moment: Make it fast, hot, and wild.
Pure nirvana: Into hair-pulling? Do it now.

87   The heart press

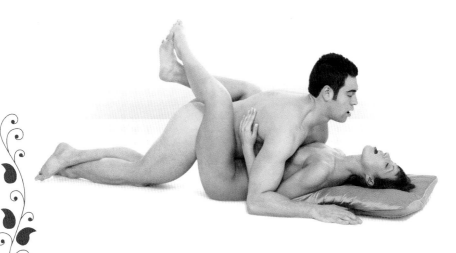

He presses his chest to hers, and she hugs him with her arms and legs.
They both cross their ankles.

Divine moment: Do it in a candlelit room.
Pure nirvana: Let your romantic side take over.

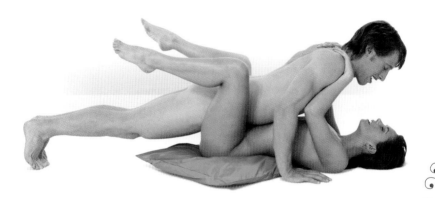

She grips him with raised thighs as he pumps on his hands and toes.

Divine moment: Slow to a trot to last a bit longer.
Pure nirvana: Admire the scenery as you go.

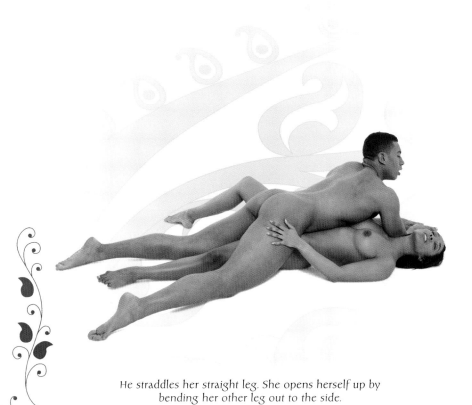

*He straddles her straight leg. She opens herself up by
bending her other leg out to the side.*

Divine moment: Do it on a PVC sheet covered in oil.
Pure nirvana: Slither your way to paradise.

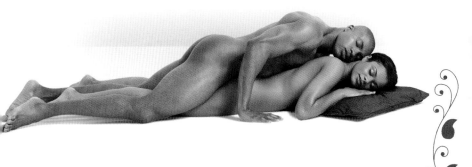

She lies on her front, and he covers her body with his,
taking his weight on his hands.

Divine moment: Girls—enjoy that sandwiched feeling.
Pure nirvana: Lie still, and flex your love muscle inside her.

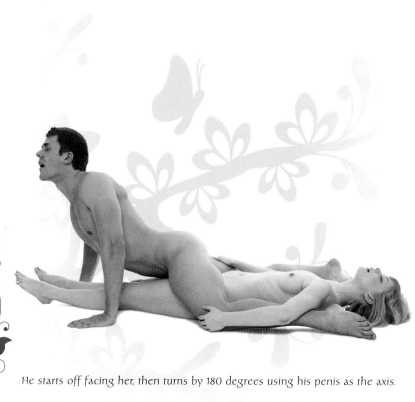

He starts off facing her, then turns by 180 degrees using his penis as the axis.

Divine moment: Girls—"embrace him around the back all the time."
Pure nirvana: If you discover bliss at 90 degrees, stay there.

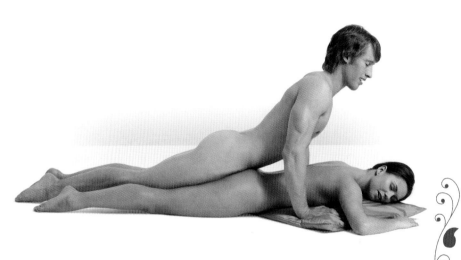

She lies flat on her tummy while he supports himself
on his arms, and penetrates from behind.

Divine moment: Work together to locate her G-spot.
Pure nirvana: Use your glans as a G-spot massage tool.

93 The rising bough

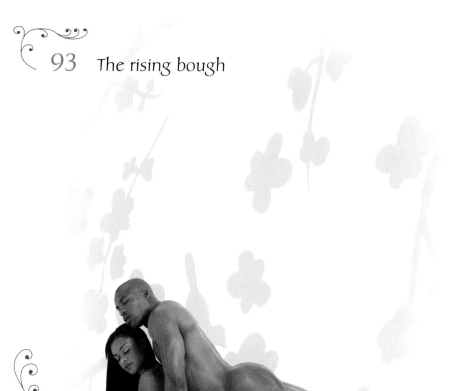

They lie with their bodies curved upward; she underneath, and he on top.

Divine moment: Re-live those teenage memories of sex in a twin-size bed.
Pure nirvana: End in doggie—so she can get a hand in.

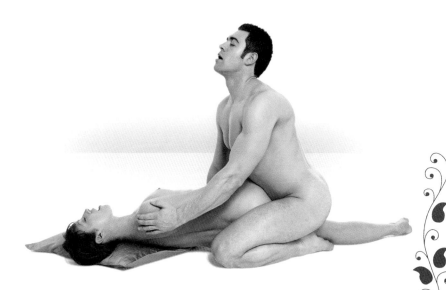

He kneels and enters as she lies in a semi-fetal position.

Divine moment: Do it first thing while the coffee's brewing.
Pure nirvana: Stroke her back before introducing your wand.

The woman of Avantika

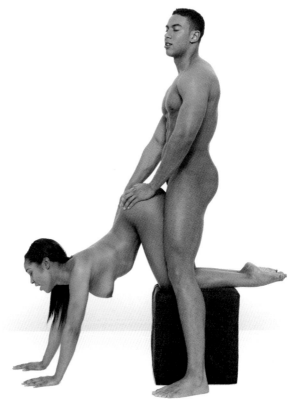

*She kneels on the edge of a block/chair, and puts her hands
on the floor, and her ass in the air.*

Divine moment: Do it in front of a full-length mirror.
Pure nirvana: Firmly grab her butt cheeks.

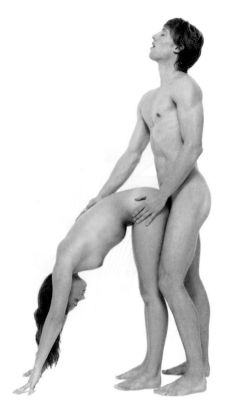

He stands and penetrates as she bends from the waist.
She puts her hands on the floor for balance.

Divine moment: Ladies—floor too far? Cheat with your hands on your knees.
Pure nirvana: Do it in the hallway as soon as you get home.

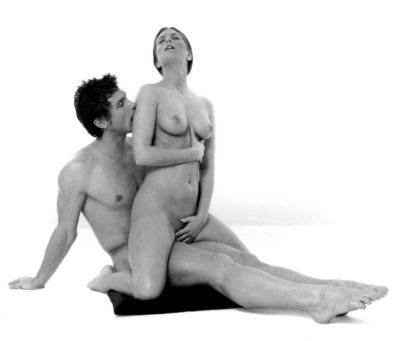

He sits with his legs stretched out, and she sits astride him.

Divine moment: Girls—do the Kegels you've been practicing.
Pure nirvana: Squeeze him hard—like "the hand that milks the cow."

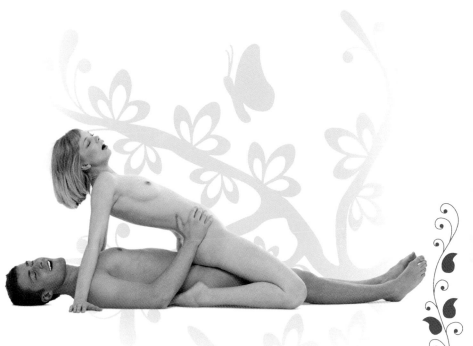

She kneels across his prone body, and leans back
so that her body is parallel to his.

Divine moment: Girls—do some rapid hip flicks on his virile member.
Pure nirvana: Guys—there's nothing to do except lie back and enjoy.

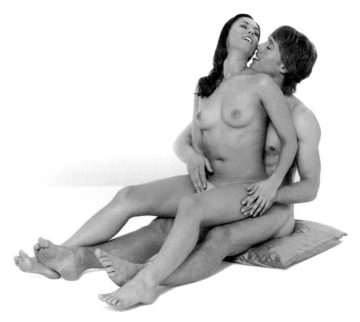

He sits against a wall, and she sits astride him fitting her body to his.

Divine moment: If it's too sedate, add buzz with a vibrator.
Pure nirvana: Make it a quickie so his legs don't die.

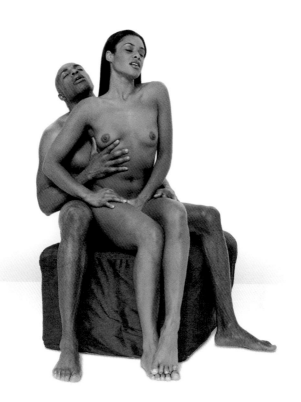

He sits on a chair, and she lowers herself onto his waiting erection.

Divine moment: Combine sex and food—do it at the dinner table.
Pure nirvana: Coat each other in something sweet and saucy.

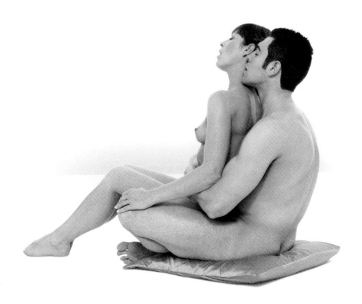

He sits cross legged, and she sits on his lingam with her back to him.

Divine moment: Use it to take a breather between more frenetic positions.
Pure nirvana: Stroke her front with your hands.

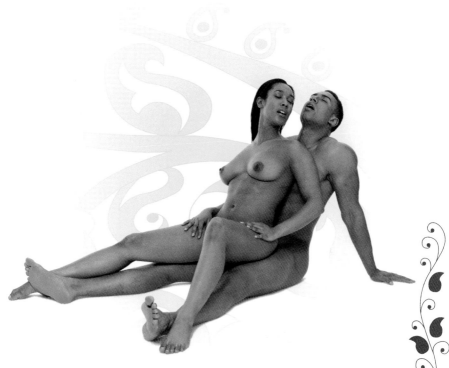

He sits back, resting on his hands. She gets on top, and encloses him.

Divine moment: Girls—lean back like you're on a sun lounger.
Pure nirvana: Try it in the back of a van on a bumpy road.

103 Mounting the throne

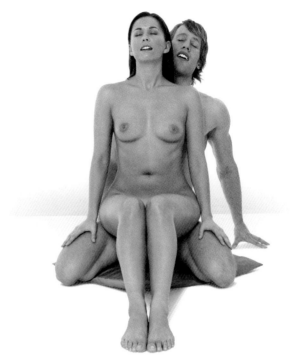

He kneels with his legs wide apart, and she slides herself on to him.

Divine moment: Offer her service by hand.
Pure nirvana: Squeeze his thighs if he's doing it right.

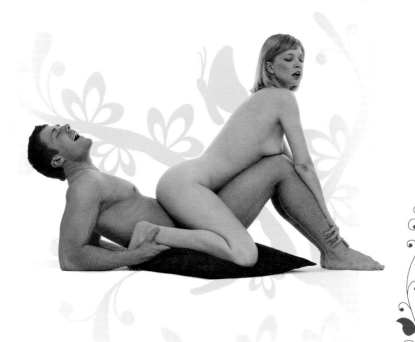

He lies back on his elbows with his knees bent. She kneels astride him,
pressing her breasts against his knees.

Divine moment: Use a spare finger to caress her back door.
Pure nirvana: Tickle his balls in return.

105 The diving swallow

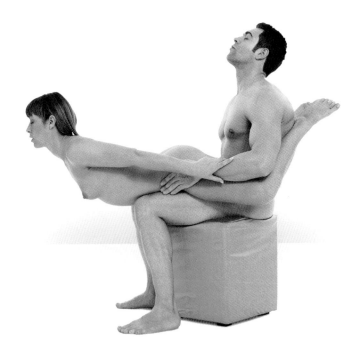

He sits on a seat, and she grips him with her thighs as she lies across his lap.

Divine moment: Stand up, and spin around the room like sexual acrobats.
Pure nirvana: Girls—put your hands on the floor when the novelty wears off.

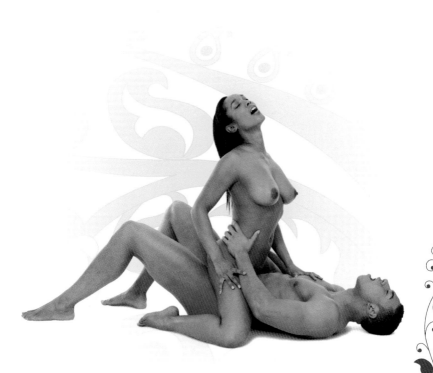

He lies back with his knees bent, and she hops on top in a kneeling position.

Divine moment: The "tongs" are your vaginal muscles—grip him hard.
Pure nirvana: Guys—ripple and flutter your muscles too.

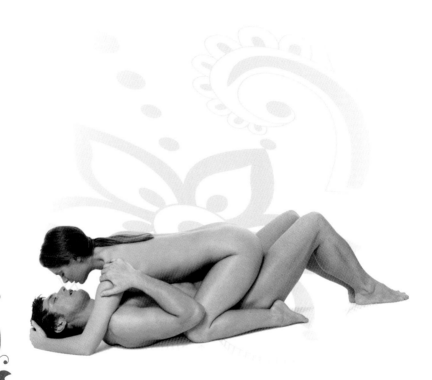

She gets on top in a kneeling position, and leans forward to rest on her elbows.

Divine moment: Say, "I was laid down by you,
I shall therefore lay you down in return."
Pure nirvana: Give him a "clasping kiss" (position 36).

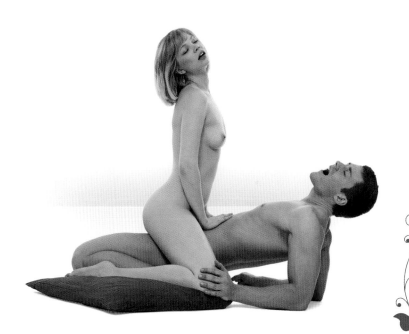

He gets into a kneeling position, and leans back on his elbows.
She kneels with her thighs around his waist.

Divine moment: Ladies—align your clitoris with his pubic bone, and ride.
Pure nirvana: Gents—stay still.

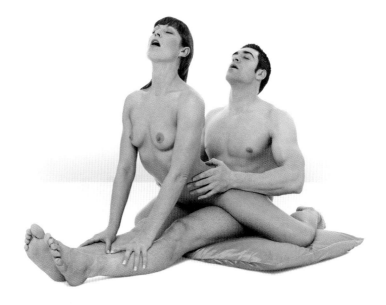

She straddles his lap with her back to him, then swings forward to lean on his calves.

Divine moment: You can't see each other's faces—abandon yourself to fantasy.
Pure nirvana: Girls—move into a squat when you want more in-out.

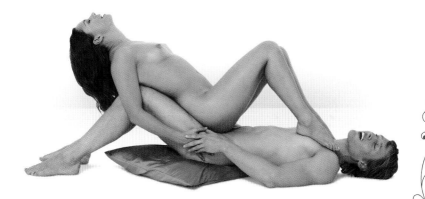

She lies back on the ramp of his thighs, and rests her feet on his chest.

Divine moment: Guys—lift your head to get a close-up.
Pure nirvana: Girls—part your knees.

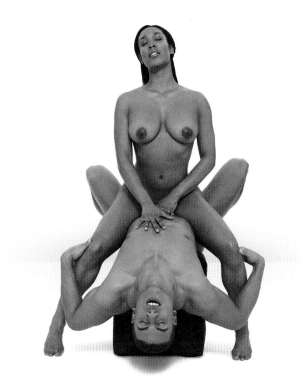

He does a backbend over a block while she sits astride him, feet on the ground.

Divine moment: Feel the union of your male and female energies.
Pure nirvana: Guys—relish the ultimate head rush.

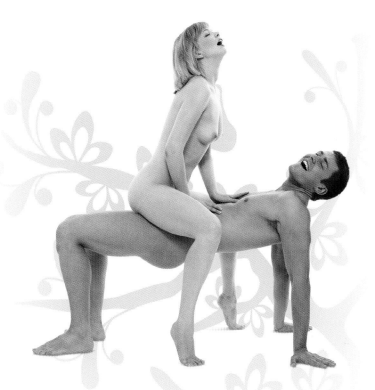

He raises himself into a platform, resting on his hands and feet, and she straddles him.

Divine moment: Make it an outdoor quickie.
Pure nirvana: Guys—feel smug and chivalrous.

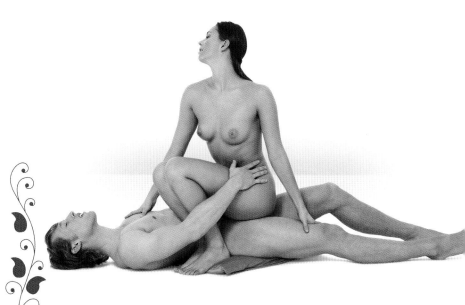

She impales herself upon him in a sitting position, and "spins" around full circle.

Divine moment: Say, "Come on baby, let's do the twist."
Pure nirvana: She moves with respect for his pole.

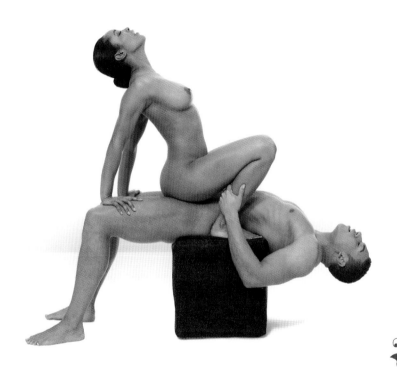

She straddles him in a sitting squat as he lies back across a block or stool.

Divine moment: She bobs and bounces from tip to base.
Pure nirvana: Do it on the edge of the bed so he's got
somewhere to lay his head.

115 The panting position

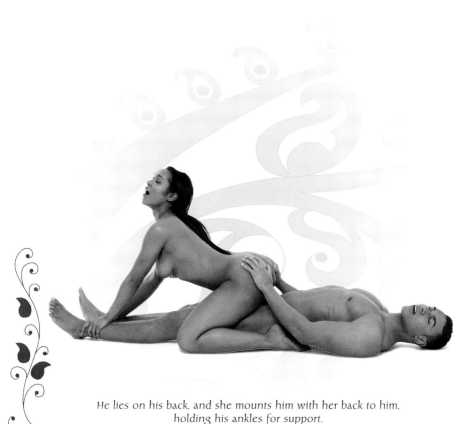

He lies on his back, and she mounts him with her back to him, holding his ankles for support.

Divine moment: She wiggles her ass from side to side.
Pure nirvana: He gives her a helping hand.

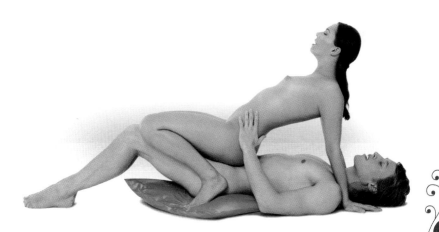

*She squats on top of him then leans back to rest on her hands
while he makes a rear entry.*

Divine moment: She discovers her G-spot.
Pure nirvana: Enhance the moment by aiming your member toward her navel.

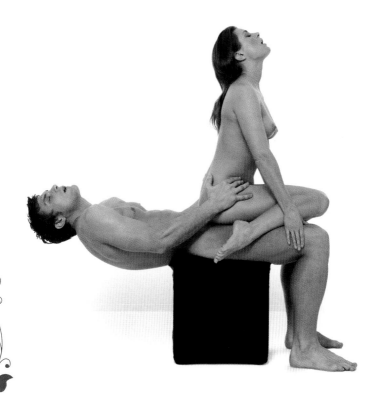

He lies back on a block while she straddles him, facing away with her knees bent.

Divine moment: You both get slick with oil or lube.
Pure nirvana: He pushes her back and forth.

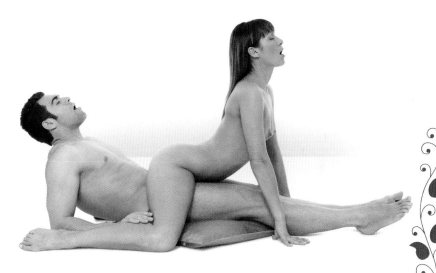

He reclines on his back while she sinks onto him on her hands and knees.

Divine moment: Explain that women of Bahlika need multiple men.
Pure nirvana: She gives mouth congress to a third party.

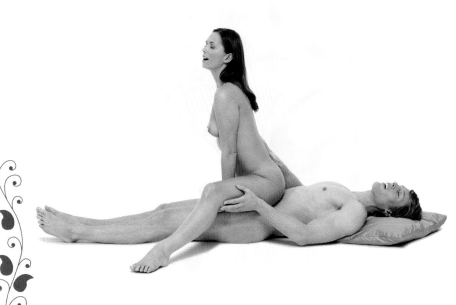

He lies flat on the ground while she sits astride him, legs spread wide.

Divine moment: Guys—stroke her back and thigh.
Pure nirvana: Girls—make it a four-hander: stroke yourself too.

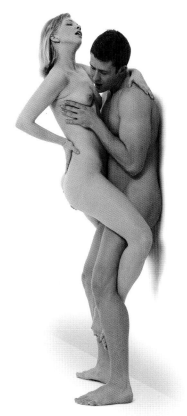

He stands with his back against a wall while she twines her legs around his.

Divine moment: Lick her nipple for the ultimate in multitasking.
Pure nirvana: Slide like butter down his legs when you
want a change of position.

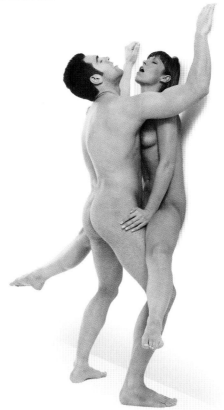

He pins her against the wall with his body, and holds her up with his thighs.

Divine moment: Do it in your private library.
Pure nirvana: Wedge her ass on a penis-height bookshelf.

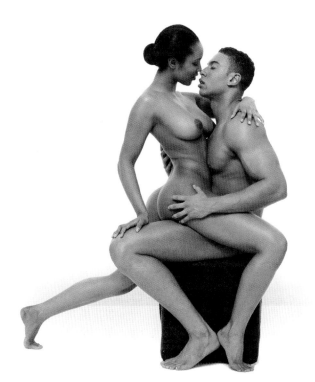

He sits in a chair, and she eases herself onto his lap—
one leg across his, and one stretched out behind.

Divine moment: Act the parts of haughty princess/horny prince...
Pure nirvana: ...or, if you prefer, princess and servant boy.

123 The silk-cotton tree

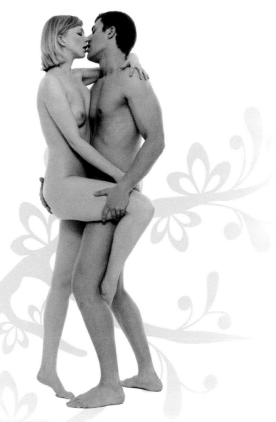

They stand facing each other, and she casually hooks one leg around his.

Divine moment: Try it during an illicit supply-closet fumble.
Pure nirvana: Make it an appetizer rather than the main course.

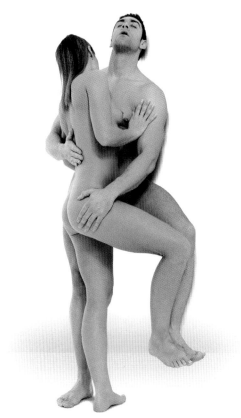

*They stand face-to-face with his back against a wall
and do a frog-style leg bend.*

Divine moment: Make life easier with a footstool.
Pure nirvana: Use it as a prime groping opportunity.

125 Yantra

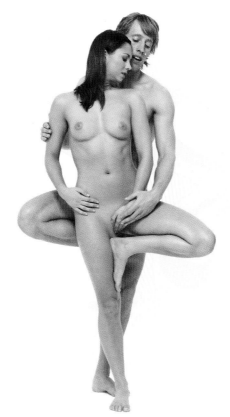

He stands behind her, and they both press a heel against their opposite thigh.

Divine moment: Photograph yourselves.
Pure nirvana: Impress everyone with your new screensaver.

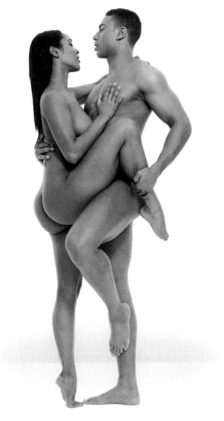

She hooks her leg over his waist while he raises a supporting thigh.

Divine moment: Delicious lusting even if he can't get it in.
Pure nirvana: Guys—go the whole nine yards and pick her up.

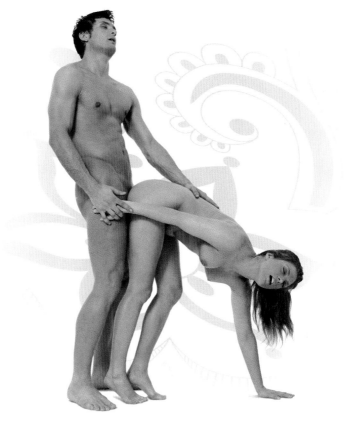

He enters her as she bends over—for support she puts one hand on the floor and one hand on his leg.

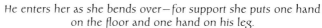

Divine moment: Let your knees buckle so you end up on the floor doggie style.
Pure nirvana: Up the sexual tension by doing it somewhere you shouldn't.

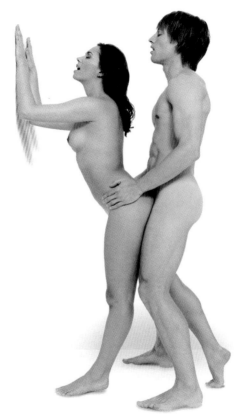

She braces herself against a firm surface, and pushes her butt out while he makes a rear entry.

Divine moment: Girls—wriggle your butt into position.
Pure nirvana: Knock gently on her backdoor.

129 Chitralekha's dream

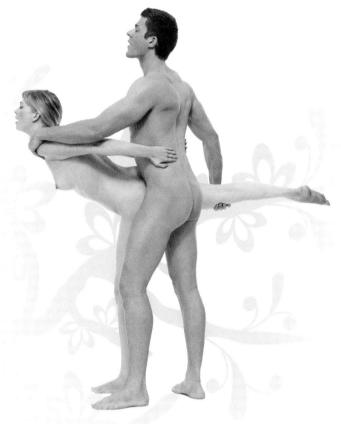

*He stands behind as she balances on one leg,
her body in a horizontal position.*

Divine moment: Conjure up your favorite "sex-while-ice-skating" fantasy.
Pure nirvana: Guys—give a good supporting act.

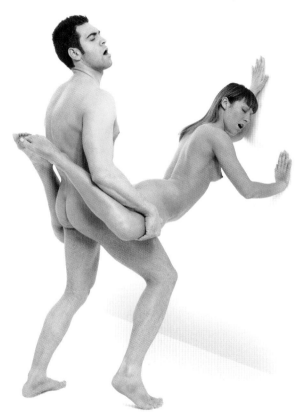

*He holds her in a wheelbarrow position as she presses
her hands against a wall.*

Divine moment: Put pillows on the floor to give her a soft landing.
Pure nirvana: Then join her down there.

131 The lotus position

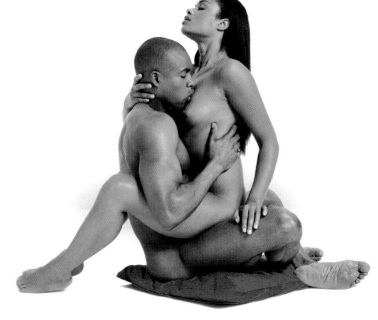

He gets into the lotus position (or crosses his legs), and she sits in his lap.

Divine moment: Find your Tantric connection.
Pure nirvana: Feel your kundalini rising.

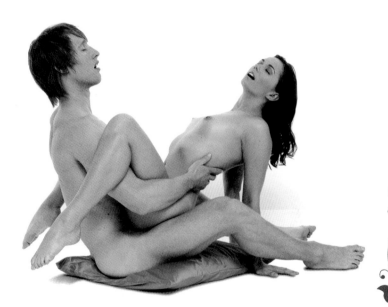

She sits in his lap, and leans back on her hands, her legs over his elbows.

Divine moment: Try it in a jacuzzi.
Pure nirvana: Enjoy the bubble and fizz.

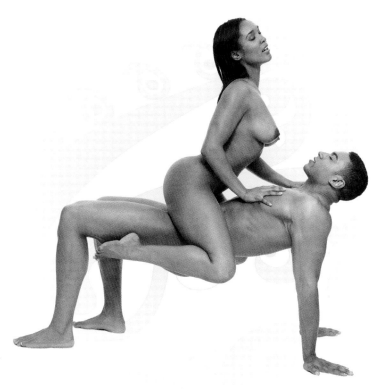

He rests, belly up, on his hands and feet while she straddles and rides.

Divine moment: Do it while she's suspended in a harness.
Pure nirvana: Have her air-lifted off when it gets too much.

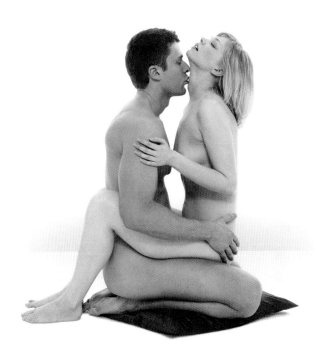

He kneels with her bottom on his lap, her legs around him,
and his lips on her neck.

Divine moment: Explore virgin territory together.
Pure nirvana: Make the build up slow and sensual.

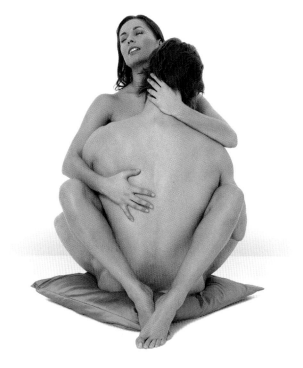

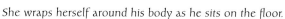

She wraps herself around his body as he sits on the floor.

Divine moment: Tenderly kiss her neck.
Pure nirvana: Rock gently as if you're in a boat.

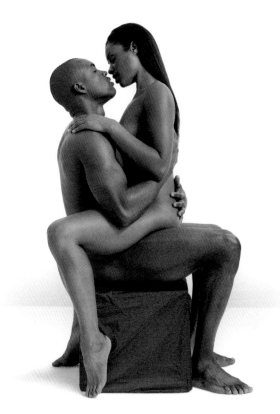

He sits in a chair, and cuddles her on his lap.

Divine moment: Feel the love.
Pure nirvana: Don't move, just kiss.

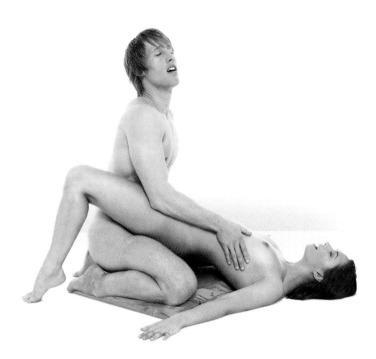

He kneels, and she clasps his waist with her thighs.

Divine moment: Invite him in by raising your hips and parting your legs.
Pure nirvana: Guys—RSVP to say you'll be coming.

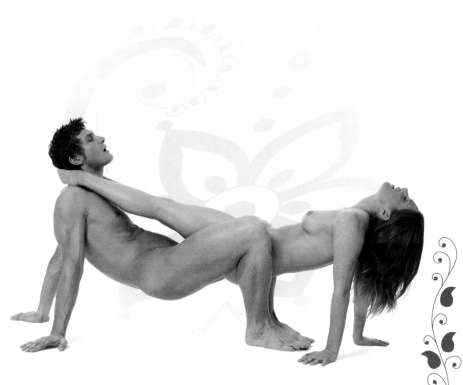

She rests her ankles on his shoulders so they make
a table shape with their bodies.

Divine moment: Thinking, "Hmmm, this is novel...."
Pure nirvana: Sink gratefully to the floor when your table starts to sag.

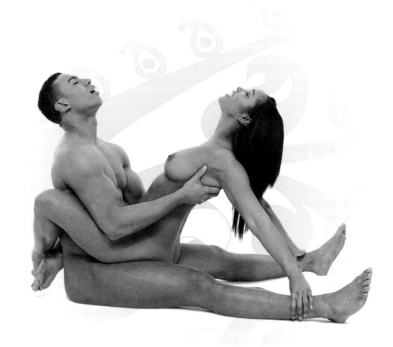

*She straddles him in a face-to-face sitting position,
then leans back to grasp his ankles.*

Divine moment: Girls—go for a sexy head-thrown-back look.
Pure nirvana: Guys—open your eyes to appreciate it.

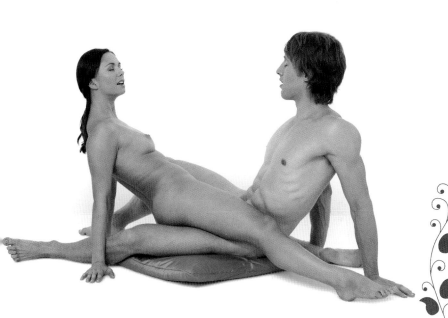

She scissors her legs through his in a sitting position.

Divine moment: Get comfy, and stay awhile.
Pure nirvana: Invent novel ways of moving.

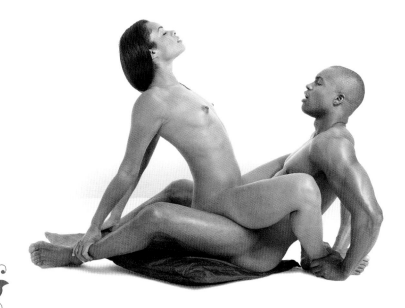

*She sits on his lap, and they both grip each other's ankles
to trap his snake inside her.*

Divine moment: Enjoy the frisson of bondage.
Pure nirvana: If the frisson amounts to a thrill, buy some bondage tape.

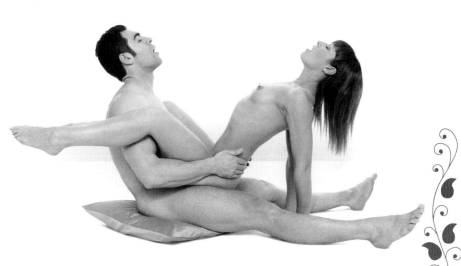

He sits on the floor, and holds her in his arms. She leans back on her hands and hooks her legs over his biceps.

Divine moment: Do what the name suggests.
Pure nirvana: Shout things you've never shouted.

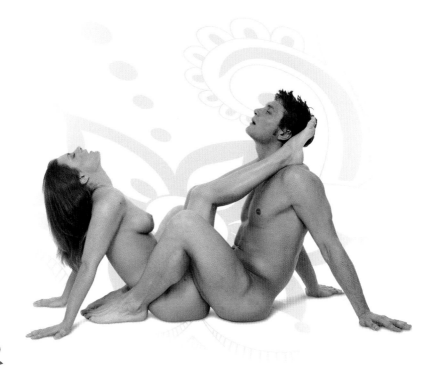

She rests her heels on his shoulders as they both lean back on their arms, buttocks pressed close.

Divine moment: Ruffle his hair with your toes.
Pure nirvana: Bump and wiggle until "the supreme moment arrives."

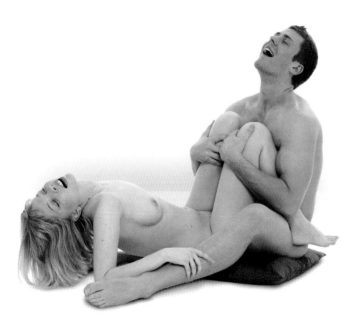

He hugs her knees to his chest, and she rests on her elbows.

Divine moment: Carefully plug yourself into her socket.
Pure nirvana: Feel the current start to flow.

145 The rising limb

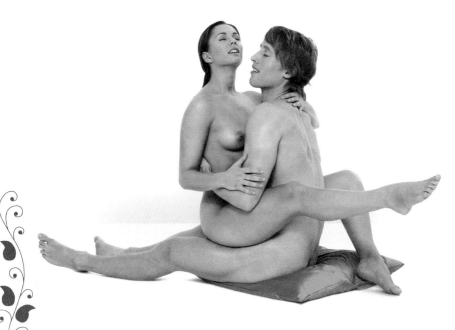

She straddles him in a sitting position—one foot on the floor, one off.

Divine moment: It's not rampant, so make it soulful.
Pure nirvana: Girls—raise your leg to find the perfect angle.

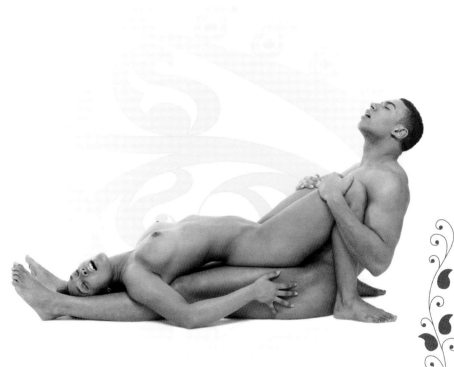

She rests her body on his thighs and her head between his calves.

Divine moment: Girls—lie back and take it easy.
Pure nirvana: Guys—move like you're rowing a boat.

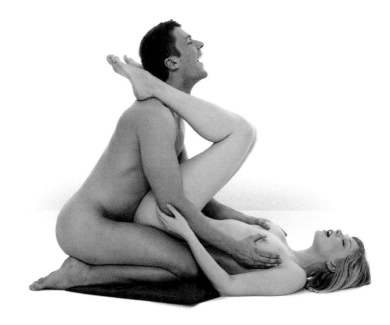

She lies on her back in a "Z" shape with her feet over his shoulders.

Divine moment: Take her nipples in hand.
Pure nirvana: Pull him in closer with your heels.

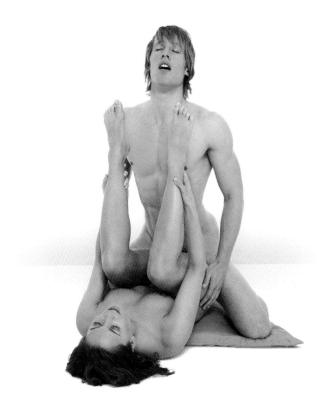

She bends her knees into her chest, and clasps her ankles as he kneels upright.

Divine moment: He gets a choice of entrance.
Pure nirvana: If he chooses the back door, bear down as he enters.

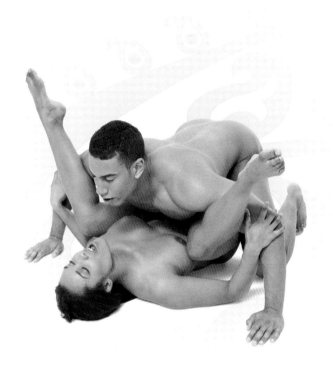

She lies underneath him with her calves resting over his arms.
He presses down upon her.

Divine moment: Girls—do a 20-minute warm-up session first.
Pure nirvana: Make this your reunion shag when you've been apart.

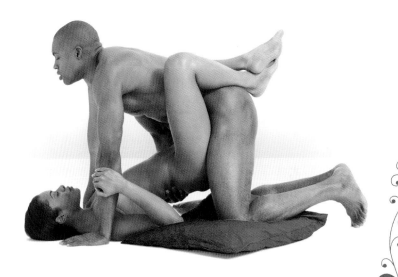

He gets on all fours, and she hangs off his waist.

Divine moment: Trap him with your legs.
Pure nirvana: Use your thigh muscles to guide him.

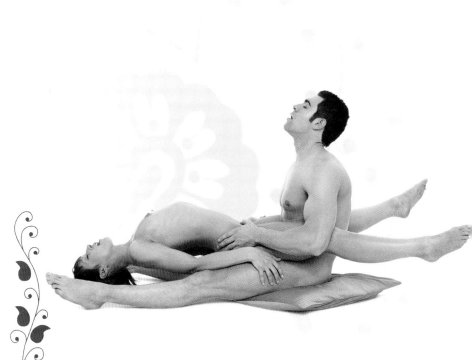

She lies on his lap so her body forms a straight line.

Divine moment: Oil each other up beforehand.
Pure nirvana: He slides her back and forth on his lap.

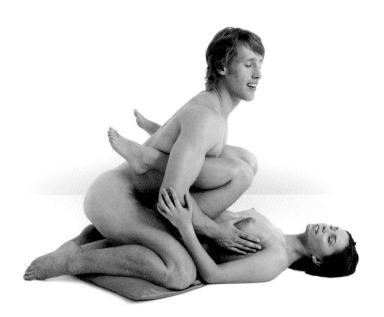

She tucks her calves under his arms, and draws her knees to her chest as he kneels and enters.

Divine moment: Ladies—press your knees together for a tight, seamless fit.
Pure nirvana: Gents—make your probing slow and gentle.

153 The refined position

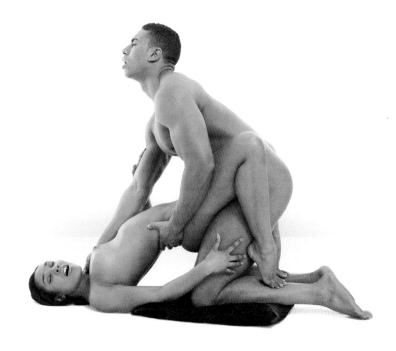

She rests her toes on his calves as she arches her back.
He kneels upright, and supports her body.

Divine moment: Enjoy the drama of throw-me-down-on-the-floor sex.
Pure nirvana: Don't just do it, *perform* it.

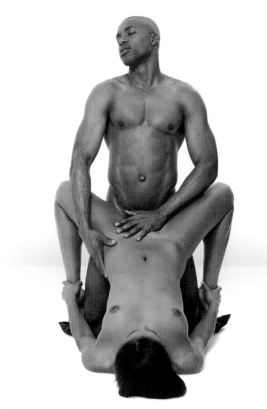

She rests on her shoulders and toes, so her body forms a bridge.

Divine moment: Press the heel of your hand against her launch pad.
Pure nirvana: Girls—shout "Yessss" at the moment of lift-off.

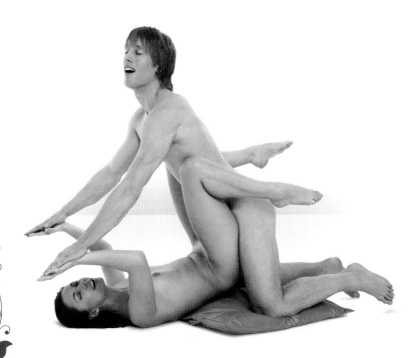

He leans forward with his palms on hers; she rests her calves on his hips.

Divine moment: Play one of those clapping games you learned in school.
Pure nirvana: High five each other afterward.

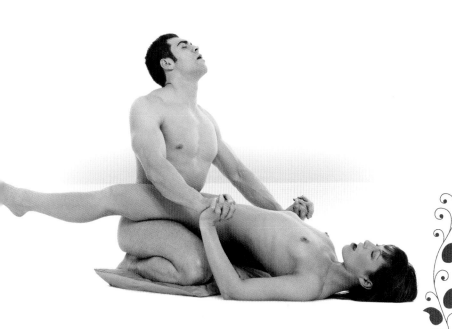

He kneels on the floor, and she lies back with her widely opened legs resting on his thighs.

Divine moment: Give him a butt massage with your heels.
Pure nirvana: Pull her up by her hands for a cuddle.

157 Star watcher

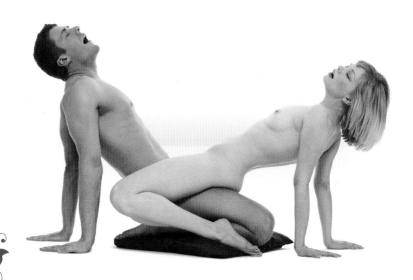

*They both kneel — she slides on top — with their heads back
and their hands behind.*

Divine moment: Do it outdoors at night.
Pure nirvana: Show her the Big Dipper.

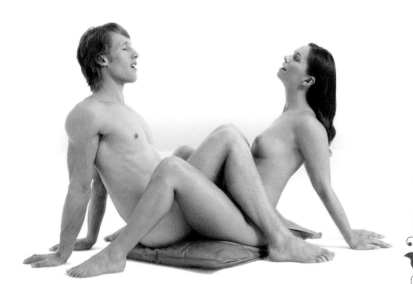

They both lean back on their arms, feet by each other's butt.

Divine moment: Think, "Well isn't this civilized?"
Pure nirvana: Nibble some canapés and sip a glass of bubbly.

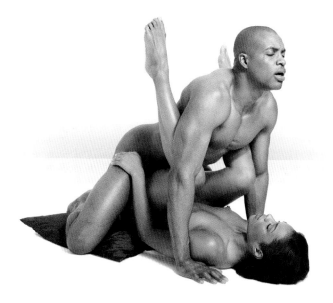

He gets on all fours, and she raises and opens her legs.

Divine moment: Do it on the living-room carpet.
Pure nirvana: Melt into the shagpile together.

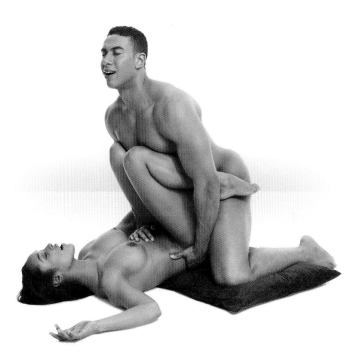

She puts her knees against his chest as she lies back and relaxes.

Divine moment: Guys—push her knees apart to get closer.
Pure nirvana: Do your best mattress-shaking, bed-breaking moves.

161 Placid embrace

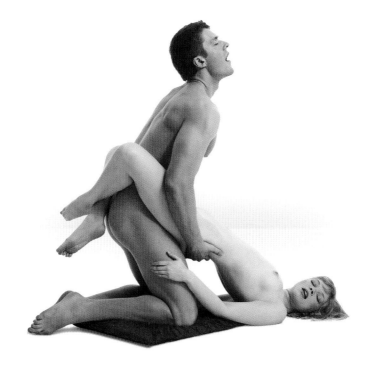

He holds the small of her back, and she wraps her legs around his waist.

Divine moment: Make it a sexy transit between standing-up
and lying-down sex.
Pure nirvana: Get a thrill from the domination/surrender vibe.

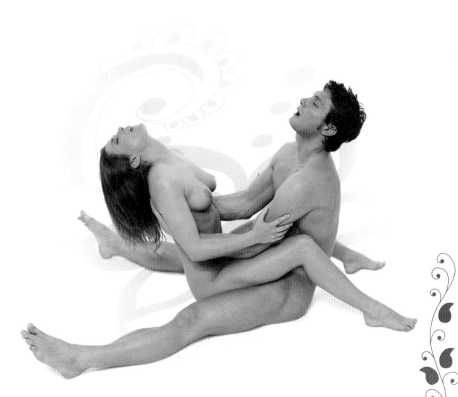

He sits with his legs out, and she nestles her ass between his thighs.

Divine moment: He closes the gaps by lifting her onto his lap.
Pure nirvana: Push against each other for the tightest connection.

163 The gaping position

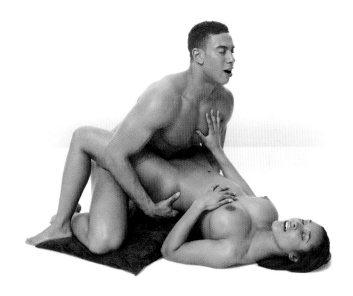

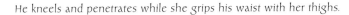

He kneels and penetrates while she grips his waist with her thighs.

Divine moment: Abandon yourself to the thrill of gotta-do-it-now sex.
Pure nirvana: Yell, "Take me, take me, yesss, ohhhhhh, yesssss."

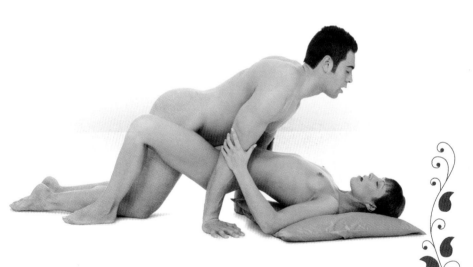

He penetrates from on top, and she raises her hips to meet him.

Divine moment: He moves down. She moves up. He moves up.
She moves down...
Pure nirvana: ...repeat as necessary.

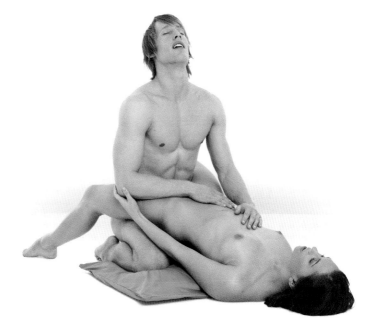

She spreads her legs wide, rests her feet on the floor, and lies back.

Divine moment: Put your white coat on—it's check-up time
(he's the gynecologist).
Pure nirvana: Measure her sensitivity in key places.

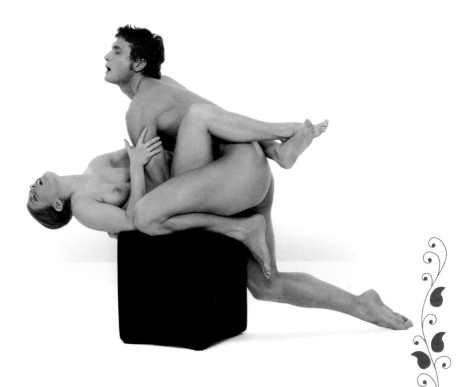

She crosses her legs behind his back as he pounces on her.

Divine moment: Do it when you're crazed with lust...
Pure nirvana: ...on the photocopier, the fire escape, the neighbors' lawn...

167 The pull of passion

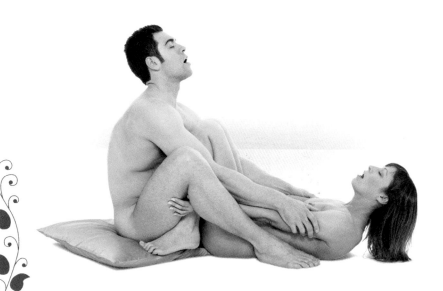

She lies back with her knees bent between his thighs.
She clasps his thighs; he clasps her arms.

Divine moment: Make it part of your morning workout.
Pure nirvana: Perfect your sit-up technique.

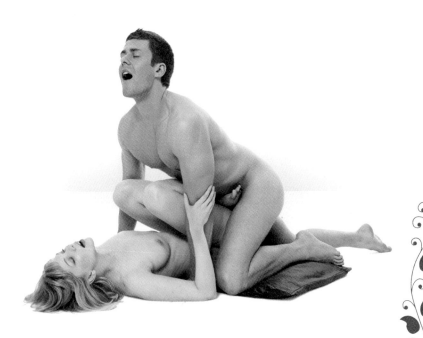

*She crosses her legs and draws them into her chest
while he penetrates from on top.*

Divine moment: Girls—use your hands to pull your knees closer to you.
Pure nirvana: Blow each other a kiss.

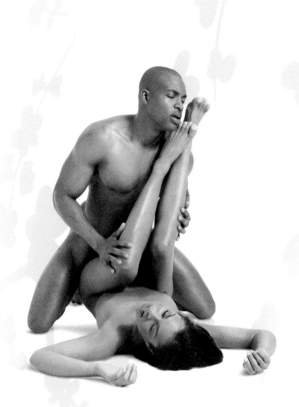

She props her feet on his shoulder as he kneels in an upright position.

Divine moment: Make it fast, hot, and urgent.
Pure nirvana: Do it while watching an x-rated movie.

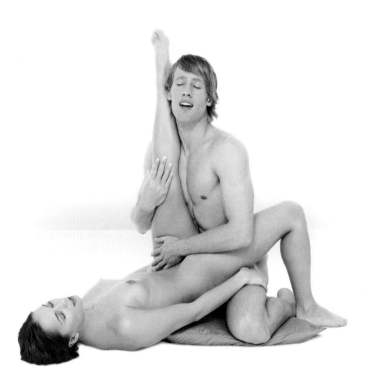

She points one leg skyward as he pushes himself between her legs.

Divine moment: Do it when she's got her leg in a cast.
Pure nirvana: Guys—keep your love limb equally stiff.

Reed in water

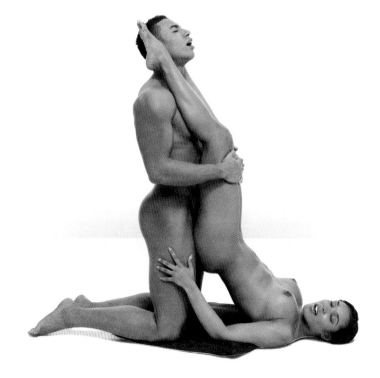

He kneels upright as she lies semi-inverted with her legs along the front of his body.

Divine moment: Use a sex wedge to get the angles right...
Pure nirvana: ...or make a pillow mountain.

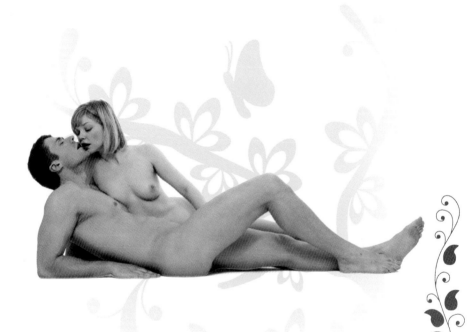

He lies back while she scratches his itch.

Divine moment: Alternate sucking with tugging.
Pure nirvana: Do it while straddling his chest.

173 Transverse lute

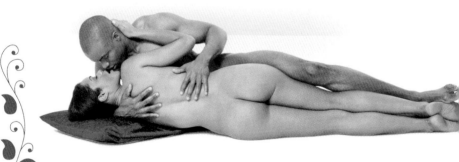

They lie facing each other on their sides, his weight supported on his elbow.

Divine moment: Feel his pathmaker trying to insinuate itself.
Pure nirvana: Assist him by opening your legs.

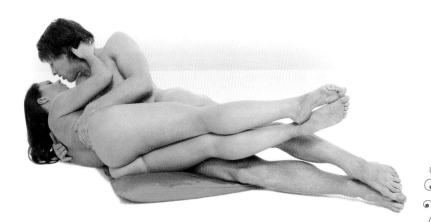

They both lie facing each other on their sides, pelvises aligned.
She raises her legs off the ground in a straight line.

Divine moment: Think, "Glad I kept up those Pilates classes."
Pure nirvana: Let your legs collapse when they start to shake.

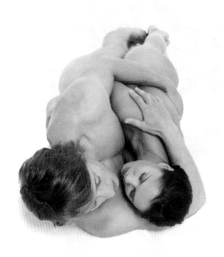

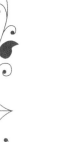

They both lie on their sides, and hug each other tight.

Divine moment: Propose marriage.
Pure nirvana: Seal it with a kiss.

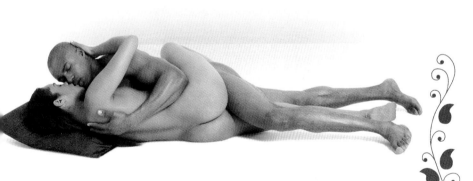

They cuddle each other in a side-by-side position, her leg around his waist.

Divine moment: Use it as a warm-up maneuver.
Pure nirvana: Get high on his thigh.

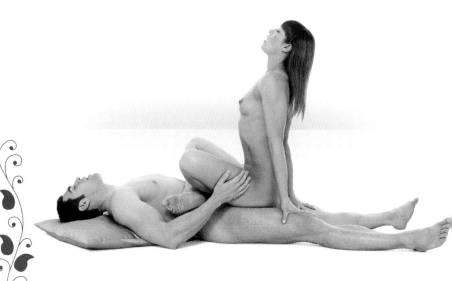

She sits cross-legged on top of his prone body.

Divine moment: Use it as your daily meditation posture.
Pure nirvana: Reach a zen-like state of bliss.

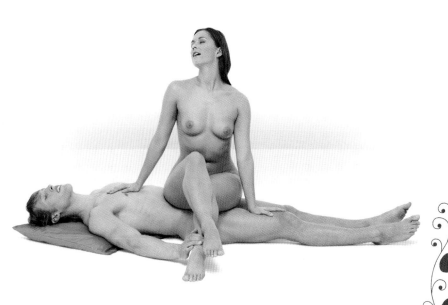

He lies flat on his back, and she encloses him side on.

Divine moment: Take him by surprise when he's stroking his oar.
Pure nirvana: Say, "You don't mind if I sit on this, do you?"

179 The inverted embrace

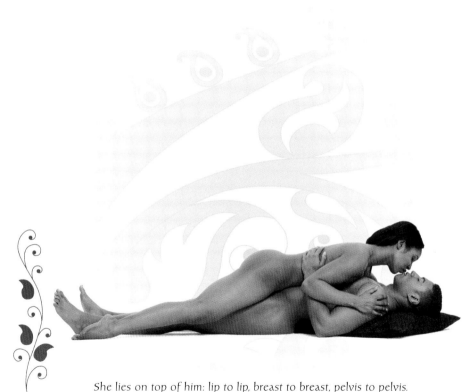

She lies on top of him: lip to lip, breast to breast, pelvis to pelvis.

Divine moment: Place him "supine on the bed or carpet,
mount his person, and satisfy your desires."
Pure nirvana: Make it the first of a woman-on-top sequence.

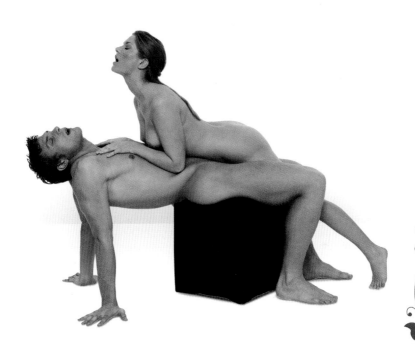

He leans back across a block while she lies between his legs.

Divine moment: Slide up and down his body.
Pure nirvana: Massage him with your breasts as you go.

181 Orgasmic role reversal

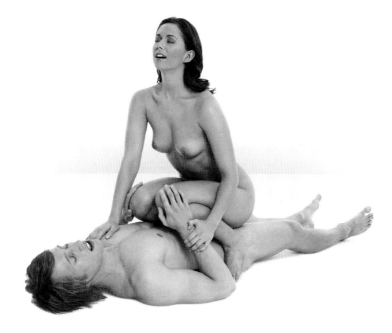

He lies flat on the bed, and she lowers herself onto him in a squat.

Divine moment: Put your hands on his manly chest...
Pure nirvana: ...now move like a rabbit.

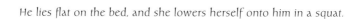

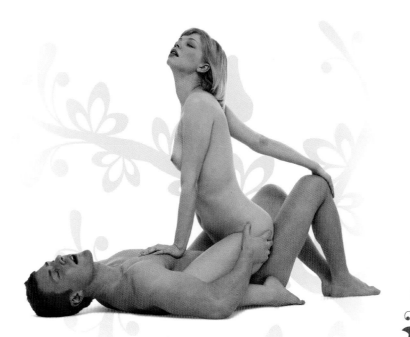

He lies on his back with his knees bent while she settles on his lingam in a semi-twist.

Divine moment: Girls—make twirling movements on his pole.
Pure nirvana: Dress code: burlesque.

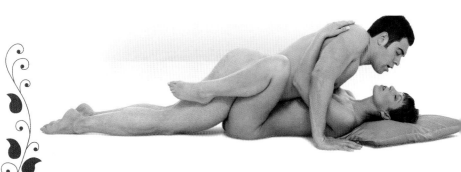

He lies on top, and she opens her legs to let him in.

Divine moment: Enjoy simple, sexy, missionary-style intimacy.
Pure nirvana: Save the fancy stuff for later.

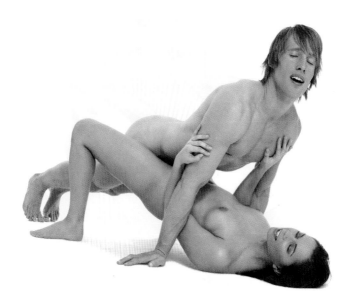

He gets into a push-up position, and she raises her pelvis to meet him.

Divine moment: Do this when you want missionary *and* maneuverability.
Pure nirvana: Girls—milk him with your movements.

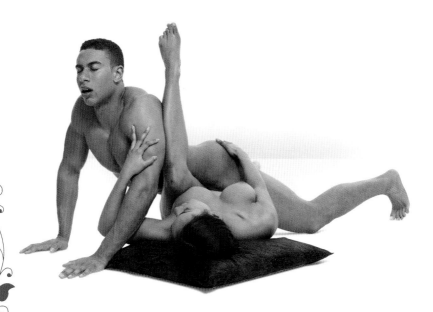

She raises one knee to her chest, and he lies diagonally across her body.

Divine moment: Guys—dip your pathfinder gently in and out.
Pure nirvana: Girls—influence his speed with your hand on his ass.

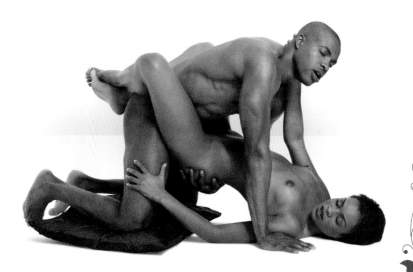

She hangs onto his body by crossing her ankles behind his back while he's on all fours.

Divine moment: Grind your organ deeply inside her.
Pure nirvana: Girls—you "may help to make the necessary movements."

187 Thighs gripping abdomen

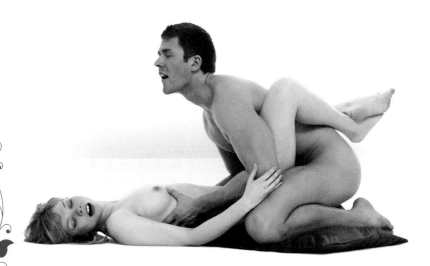

He kneels with his legs on either side of her hips.

Divine moment: Widen your legs, and pull her firmly onto you.
Pure nirvana: Cup her breasts, and massage her nipples with your thumbs.

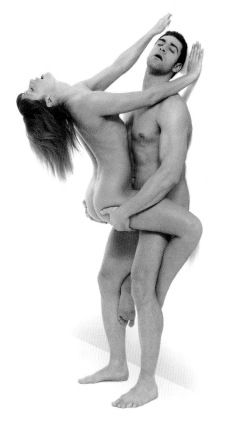

He picks her up, and she twines her legs around his as he leans against a wall.

Divine moment: Girls—grip his ivory tower.
Pure nirvana: Guys—bounce your butt against the wall.

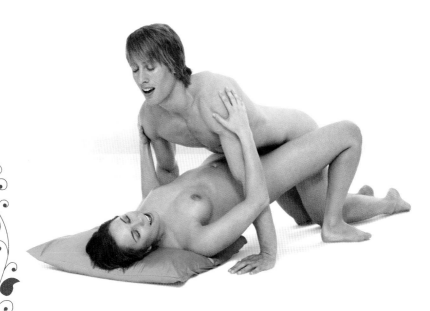

He gets on his hands and knees, and she raises her pelvis to meet him.

Divine moment: Girls—"drop your buttocks in short, sharp jerks."
Pure nirvana: Guys—"keep close, and make sure that your member
is not withdrawn."

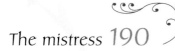

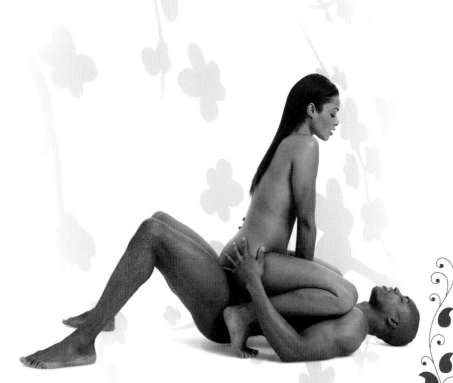

She squats on top of him as he lies on his back with his knees bent.

Divine moment: Girls—you're in charge.
Pure nirvana: Blindfold him so he doesn't know what's coming.

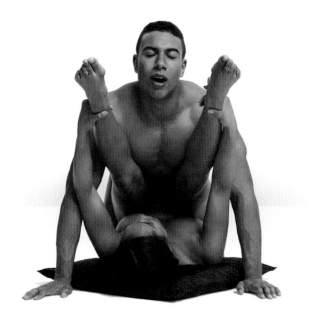

She raises her legs, and he flattens them against her body as he enters.

Divine moment: Guys—dip in with swift, shallow moves.
Pure nirvana: Thrust vigorously until your cup overflows.

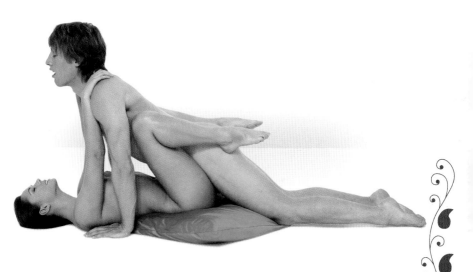

He lies on top with his arms straight, and she wraps him in her arms and legs.

Divine moment: Girls—set the pace with heel power.
Pure nirvana: Guys—wear a vibrating ring on your jade stalk.

193 The stopperage

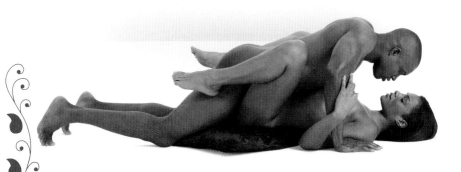

She bends her knees and raises her legs as he lies on top.

Divine moment: Girls—draw your knees to your chest
"so your vulva stands out like a sieve."
Pure nirvana: Guys—"plunge your member between her thighs."

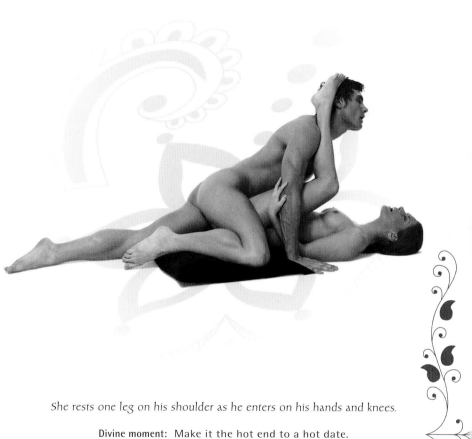

She rests one leg on his shoulder as he enters on his hands and knees.

Divine moment: Make it the hot end to a hot date.
Pure nirvana: Then spend the night together.

195 The inversion

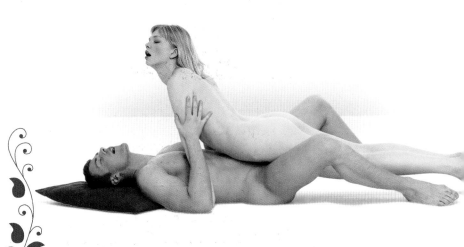

He lies on his back and opens his legs, and she climbs on top.

Divine moment: Girls—keep your legs closed for a tight, snug fit.
Pure nirvana: Try rolling over, still joined.

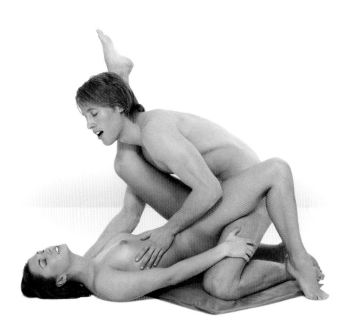

He enters in a semi-kneeling position as she stretches one leg over his shoulder.

Divine moment: Rub your member across the tip of her clitoris.
Pure nirvana: Keep going until her cloud bursts.

197 Sacred arch

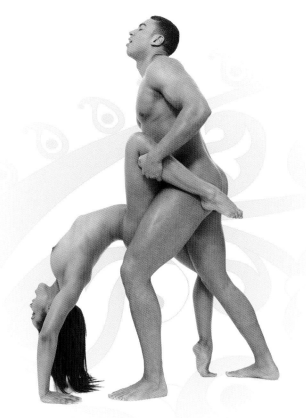

She does a backbend, and hooks one leg over his thigh.

Divine moment: Line up some spectators beforehand.
Pure nirvana: Girls—you're not dressed without nipple tassels.

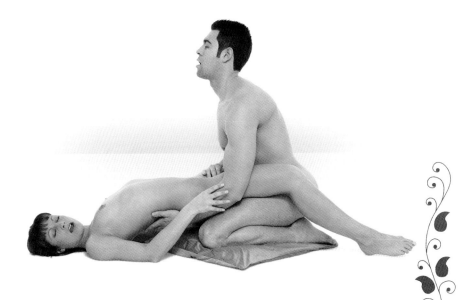

She parts her legs on his lap as he kneels on the floor.

Divine moment: Try some digital play first.
Pure nirvana: When she's ready, slip your foot in her sock.

199 Nefzawi's knot

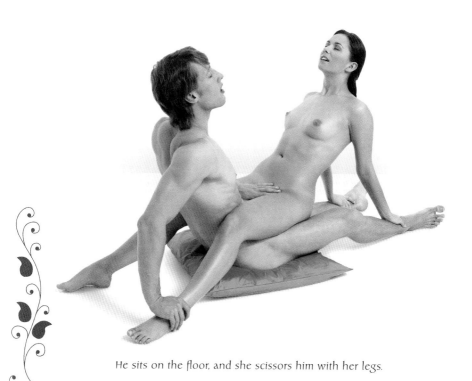

He sits on the floor, and she scissors him with her legs.

Divine moment: Show off your vibrating thumb skills.
Pure nirvana: Don't stop until she's limp with pleasure.

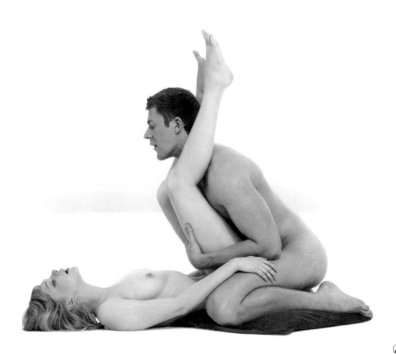

He kneels before her with her legs resting along the front of his body.

Divine moment: "Arrange the woman so your member
is exactly opposite her vulva."
Pure nirvana: "Lift her slightly—this is the moment to introduce your member."

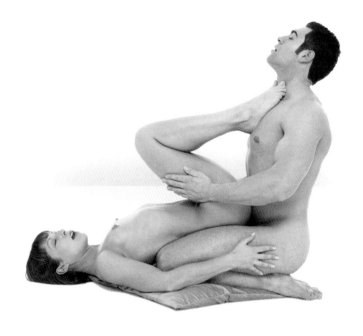

She rests her feet on his neck, and presses herself tightly between his legs.

Divine moment: Let your sword rest quietly in her sheath before you move.
Pure nirvana: Tickle his chin with your toes.

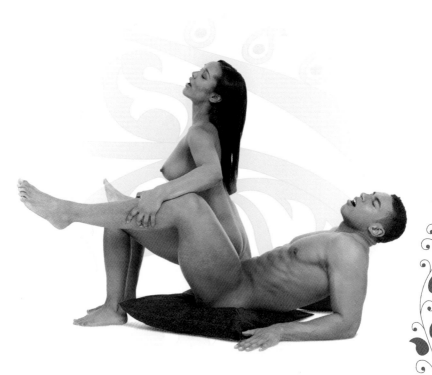

She sits astride him, and rests her forearms on his raised legs.

Divine moment: Raise yourself to delight in the perfection of her form.
Pure nirvana: Lean back, and lash him with your long hair.

203 The courageous position

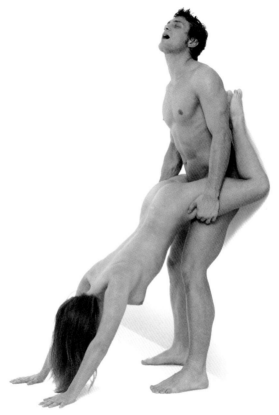

He presses himself between her legs while she inverts herself against a wall.

Divine moment: Feel your heart pumping and your limbs trembling.
Pure nirvana: Guys—stand and deliver.

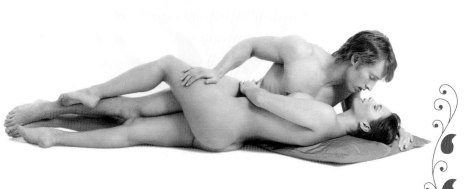

They both lie on their sides, and she hooks her upper leg over his.

Divine moment: "Penetrate her when her lips redden
and her sighs are profound."
Pure nirvana: "Clasp her, suck her, bite her, and strain her to you."

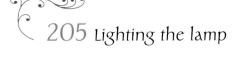

205 Lighting the lamp

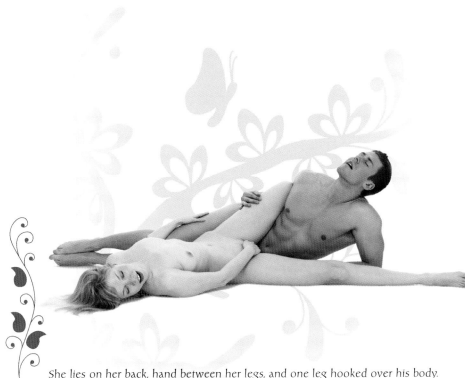

She lies on her back, hand between her legs, and one leg hooked over his body.

Divine moment: Offer to be her human dildo...
Pure nirvana: ...while she does the two-fingered shuffle.

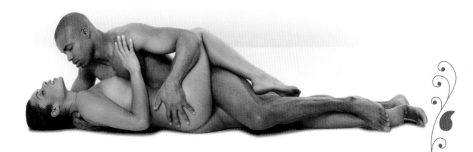

He slides his thigh between hers as they embrace on their sides.

Divine moment: "Plant a kiss on each other's moist and ardent lips."
Pure nirvana: Then quickly follow with the introduction of your member.

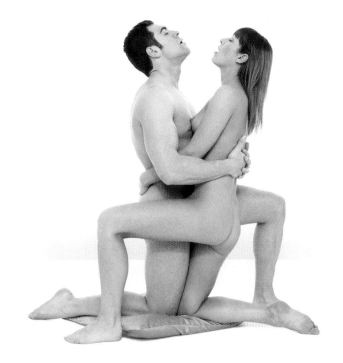

Facing, they mirror each other's posture—outer leg bent at the knee.

Divine moment: Pull him close to feel your nipples brush against his chest.
Pure nirvana: Rub your member against her pearl of heavenly delight.

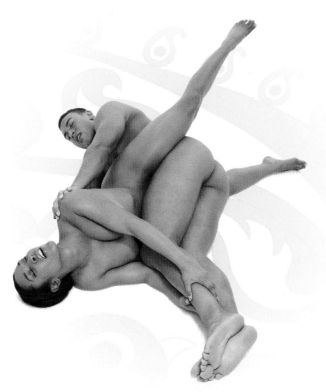

She lies on her side, and encloses him with her thighs while facing his feet.

Divine moment: Get into a sexy tangle as you figure out how to do it.
Pure nirvana: Enjoy the new spin on rear-entry.

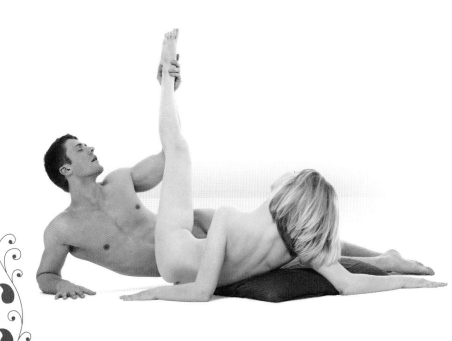

She extends her right leg to one side, and — with his aid —
extends her left to the sky.

Divine moment: Caress her shapely ankle.
Pure nirvana: Keep your leg straight to ensure free-flowing sexual energy.

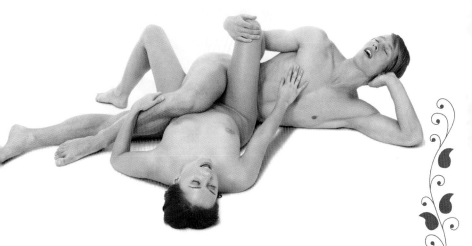

She lies on her back, and he lies on his side. He puts his top leg between hers.

Divine moment: Tilt your pelvis up to meet his thigh.
Pure nirvana: Slide your thigh along her pleasure zone.

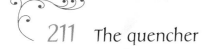

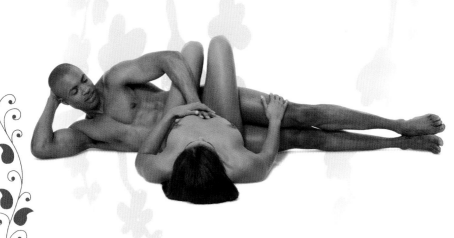

He penetrates while lying on his side at right angles to her body.

Divine moment: Make it lazy weekend sex.
Pure nirvana: Girls—adjust the fit by putting your feet on a nearby wall.

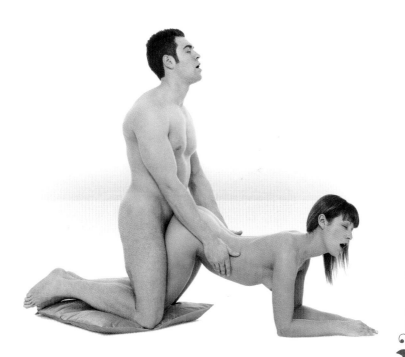

He kneels upright, and she rests on her forearms and knees.

Divine moment: Do it when you're on borrowed time.
Pure nirvana: Guys—move fast; girls—put your finger on the button.

213 The hot iron

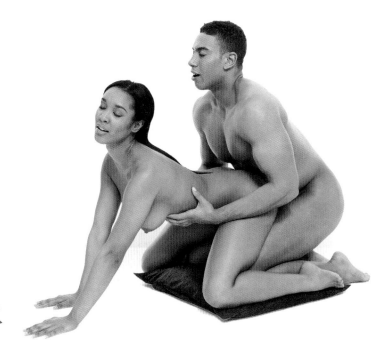

She gets on all fours, and he pulls her butt into his lap.

Divine moment: Use it to take a breather from the sixth posture (see 212).
Pure nirvana: Make sure she's sitting comfortably.

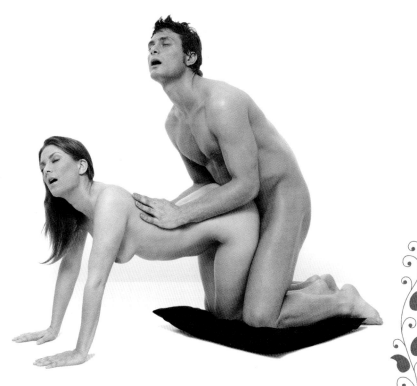

She rests on all fours with her legs together, and he kneels upright behind her.

Divine moment: Exploit the anonymity.
Pure nirvana: Think about that cute waiter/cashier/handyman.

215 The magnetic one

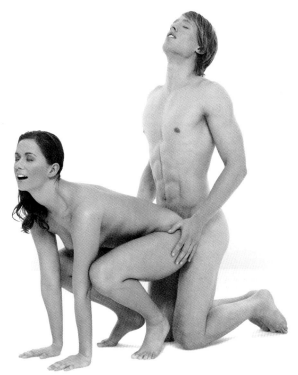

She squats with her ass raised, and he kneels and enters.

Divine moment: Try traveling along the narrow path.
Pure nirvana: Drive slowly and carefully.

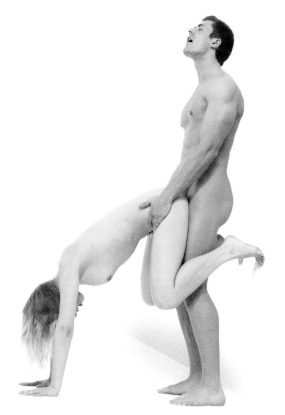

He stands, and she balances with her feet against a wall.

Divine moment: Say, "Bet your last girlfriend couldn't do this."
Pure nirvana: Enjoy the head rush.

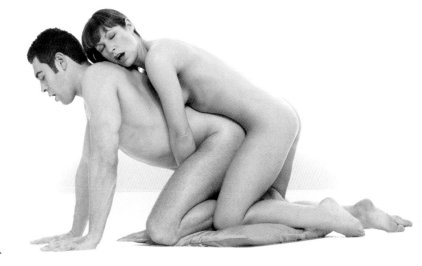

He gets on all fours, and she moulds her body to his.

Divine moment: Manhandle his lingam...
Pure nirvana: ...while pumping from behind with a strap-on.

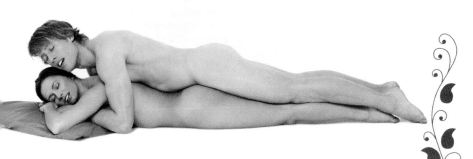

She lies on her tummy, and he covers her with his body.

Divine moment: Offer to be her human blanket.
Pure nirvana: Guys—take your weight on your elbows.

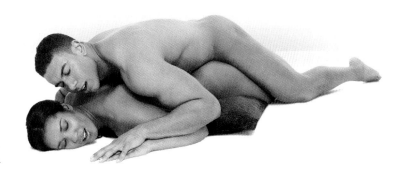

She lies on her tummy, and he climbs on top with his legs either side of hers.

Divine moment: Girls—indulge in a "being taken" fantasy.
Pure nirvana: Guys—press your hands on top of hers.

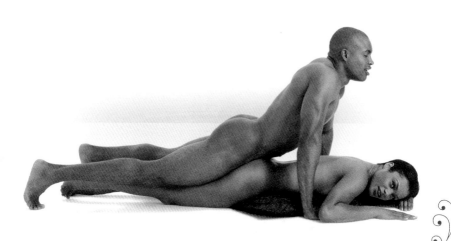

She's on her front, and he lies on top in a push-up position.

Divine moment: Guys—move your hips like Elvis.
Pure nirvana: Girls—lie on your hand for extra friction.

221 The jingler

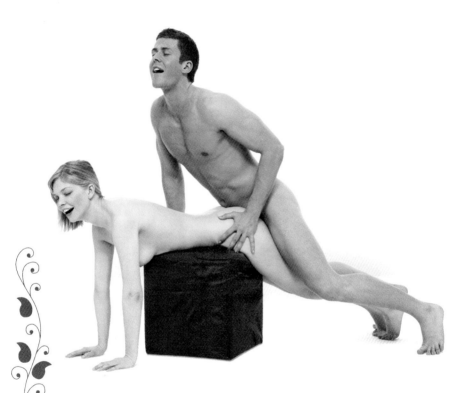

She drapes herself over a stool, and he penetrates her from behind.

Divine moment: Spank the side of her butt.
Pure nirvana: Girls—let your whole body go limp.

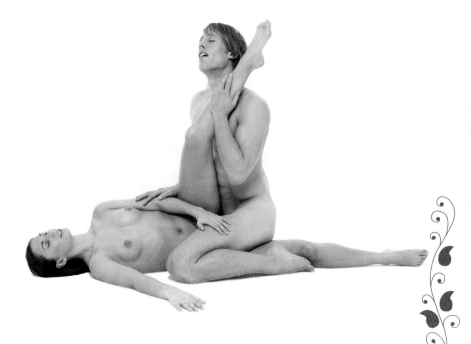

She lies on her back with one leg across his front and the other between his legs.

Divine moment: Be her personal trainer.
Pure nirvana: Do some serious groin stretching.

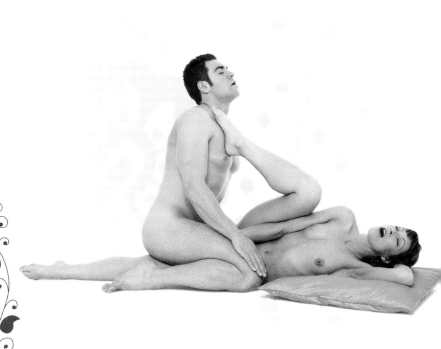

She lies on her side and plants her foot squarely on his chest.

Divine moment: Use your raised leg as a barrier to entry.
Pure nirvana: Now slowly lift the barrier.

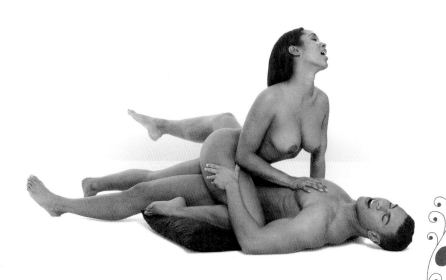

He lies on his back with his knee raised. She mounts him in a half straddle.

Divine moment: Do it on a pool table.
Pure nirvana: Say, "Can I scratch your eight-ball?"

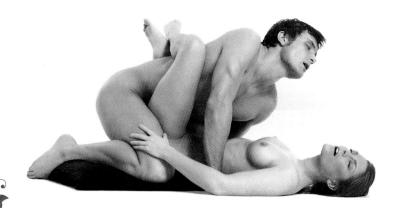

He lays her on the ground, and leans over her as she wraps her legs around his body.

Divine moment: Make it the climax of a long seduction campaign.
Pure nirvana: Make sure she comes first.

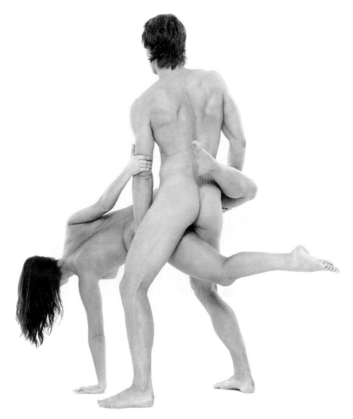

He holds her perpendicular to his body and she balances on one arm.

Divine moment: Do a dry run first.
Pure nirvana: Practice landing safely.

227 The high sprinkler

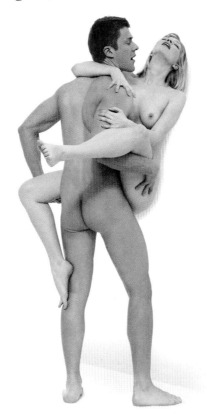

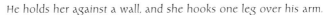

He holds her against a wall, and she hooks one leg over his arm.

Divine moment: Make it the opener to a dirty weekend.
Pure nirvana: Fall onto the hotel bed, and continue.

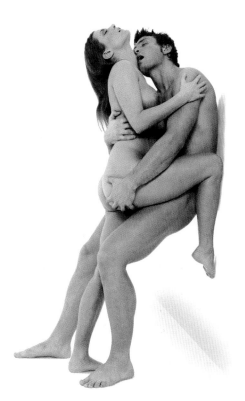

He leans against a wall, and she hooks one leg over his hip.

Divine moment: Graduate to it from an intense snog.
Pure nirvana: Get a should-we-be-doing-this-here high?

229 Frog fashion

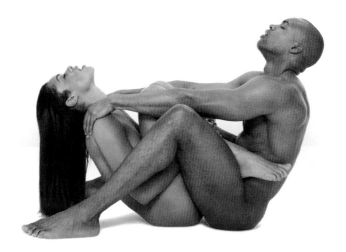

They sit opposite each other with their knees bent; his legs enclosing her body.

Divine moment: Rock and roll together.
Pure nirvana: Do it to music.

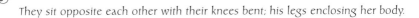

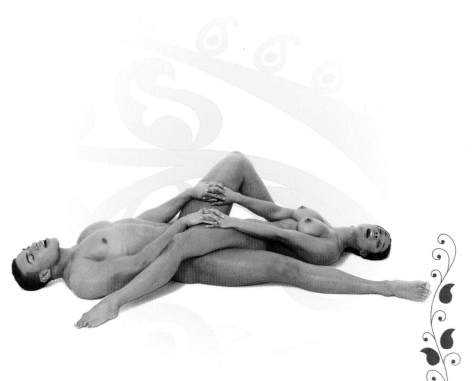

They lie on their backs, heads close to each other's feet.

Divine moment: Do the sweet holding-hands thing.
Pure nirvana: Treat it as a rest before your final destination.

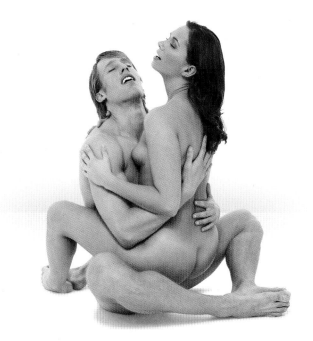

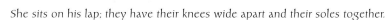

She sits on his lap; they have their knees wide apart and their soles together.

Divine moment: "Indulge in a see-saw motion, leaning backward and forward alternately."
Pure nirvana: "Take care that your movements are well-timed."

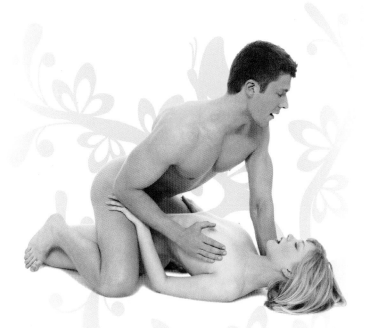

She lies back with her feet under her bottom, and he kneels astride her.

Divine moment: Girls—feel a taut stretch in your thighs.
Pure nirvana: Guys—penetrate slowly to "awaken the sucking power of her vagina."

233 The member reversed

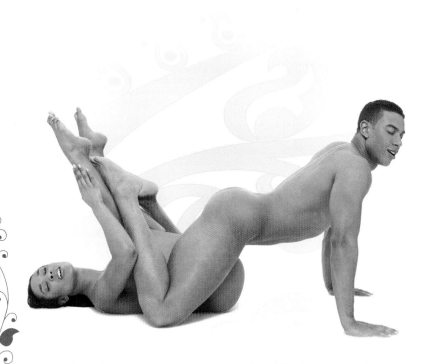

She pulls her legs up to her chest, and uses his feet to extend them over her head.

Divine moment: Admire your man's buttocks as he thrusts.
Pure nirvana: Guys—use this position to work on your upper body strength.

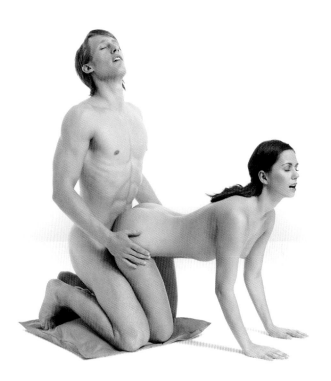

She goes on all fours, with legs slightly apart, and he takes her from behind.

Divine moment: Girls—present yourself to him in this position first.
Pure nirvana: Be self-voyeurs—watch yourselves in a mirror.

235 The announcement

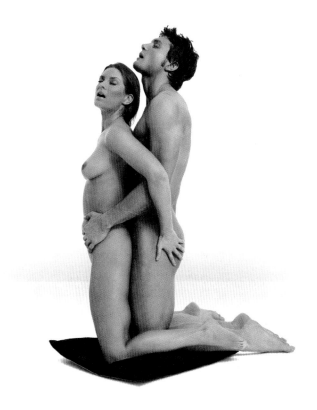

He kneels behind her with his hands on her belly.

Divine moment: Announce your arousal by pressing it into her back.
Pure nirvana: Get her up to speed with some skilled hand action.

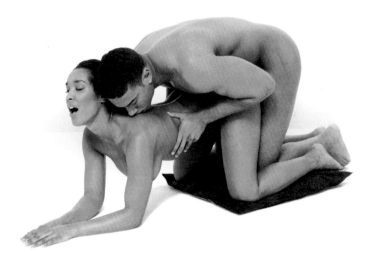

She rests on her knees and forearms while he folds himself over her.

Divine moment: Kiss her neck/ears/shoulders/back.
Pure nirvana: It's doggie plus love—enjoy it.

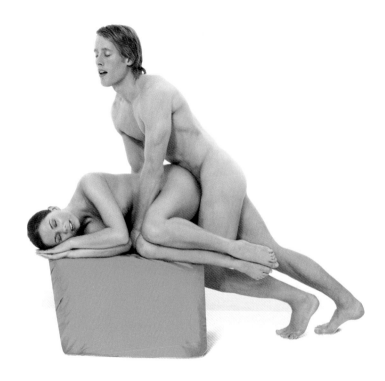

She lies on her side with her knees drawn up, and he leans over her.

Divine moment: Feign sleep so he makes all the moves.
Pure nirvana: Pull your knees to your chest to accommodate him.

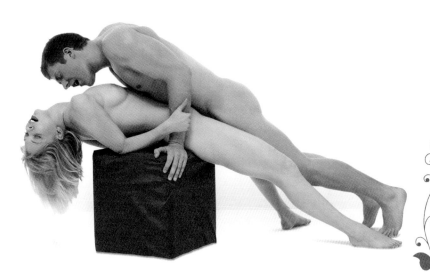

She leans back on the edge of a bed or chair, and he presses himself into her.

Divine moment: Throw her on the bed with urgent, breathy passion.
Pure nirvana: Pretend you're in a 1940s Hollywood movie.

239 The erotic repose

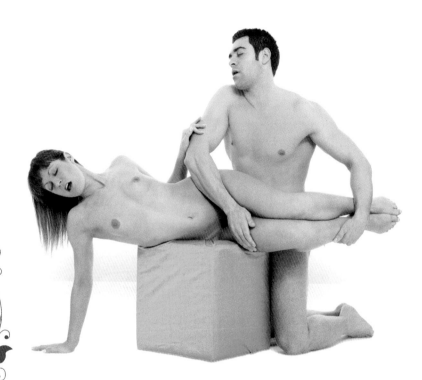

She lies on her side on a cushion or bed, and he kneels behind her.

Divine moment: Pull her amorously to the edge of the bed.
Pure nirvana: "Plunge your member to the bottom of her vagina."

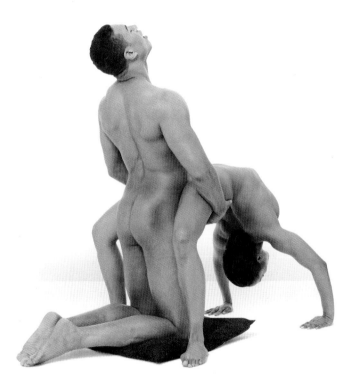

She balances on her hands and feet in an arch; he kneels between her legs.

Divine moment: Do it instead of morning yoga.
Pure nirvana: Get into it via a somersault (for sexcrobats only).

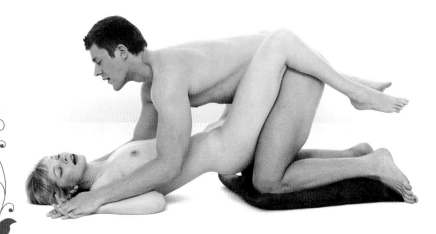

Kneeling he pulls her onto his member, then lowers her to the ground.

Divine moment: Feel aroused by her writhing within the cage of your arms.
Pure nirvana: "Know that the woman will not feel her desires satisfied, and will not love her rider unless he is able to act up to her womb."

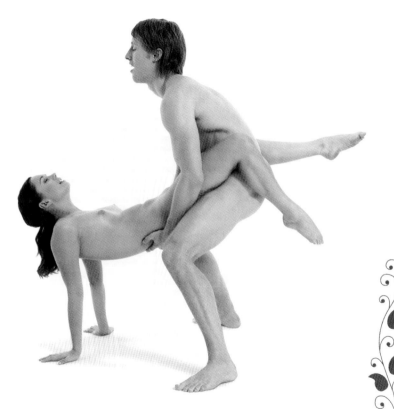

She balances on her hands facing upwards and he holds her waist.

Divine moment: Do it because there's nowhere to lie down.
Pure nirvana: Concentrate on staying connected.

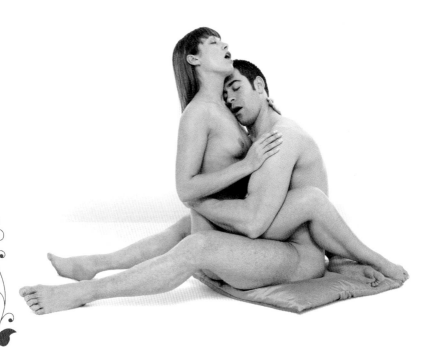

She sits in his lap with her arms and legs twined around him.

Divine moment: Cuddle as if you're trying to stay warm.
Pure nirvana: But give each other goosebumps, too.

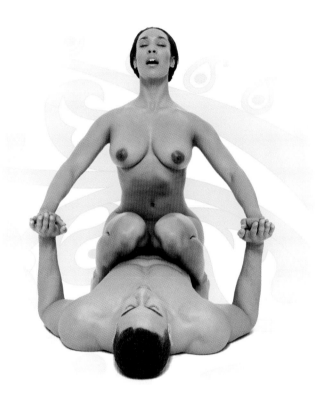

She straddles his prone body, and they press their palms together.

Divine moment: Girls—rock, sway, shuffle, grind, and bounce.
Pure nirvana: Guys—lie back and enjoy the ride.

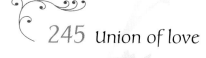

245 Union of love

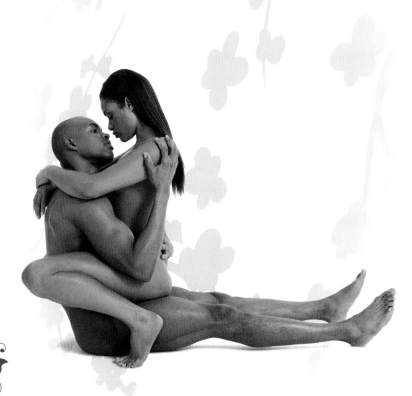

He sits with his legs straight as she squats and cuddles him.

Divine moment: Make it anniversary sex.
Pure nirvana: Whisper loving words.

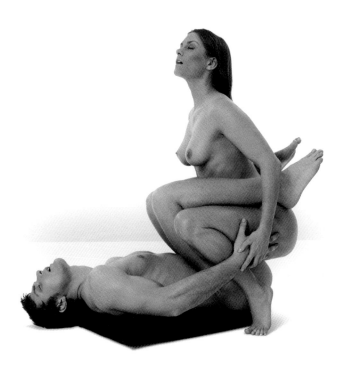

He draws his thighs up to his chest, and then she sits down,
impaling herself on his member.

Divine moment: Ride him like a stallion.
Pure nirvana: "She must not lie down, but keep seated as if on horseback."

247 The imprisoned member

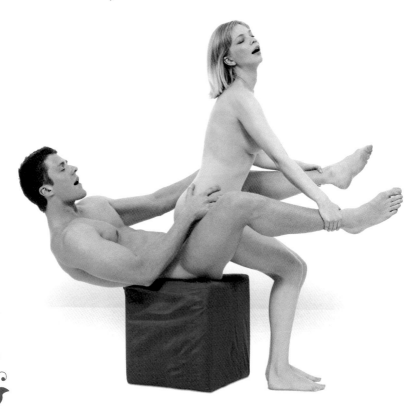

He lies back on a raised surface; she holds his legs, and sits between them.

Divine moment: Grab his ankles, and cross them in front of you.
Pure nirvana: Tell him there's no escape until you're done.

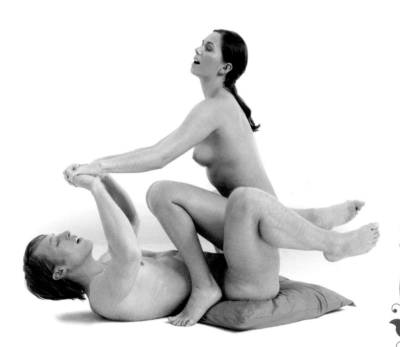

He lies on his back, knees raised, and she squats on top.

Divine moment: Invite her to straddle your saddle.
Pure nirvana: Ride him fast to the finishing line.

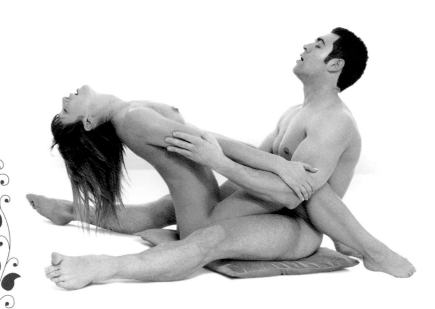

They both sit on the floor facing each other; she puts her legs
around his waist, and they both lean back.

Divine moment: Start in this position if he has a tall tower.
Pure nirvana: Girls—wiggle closer to fit more of it in.

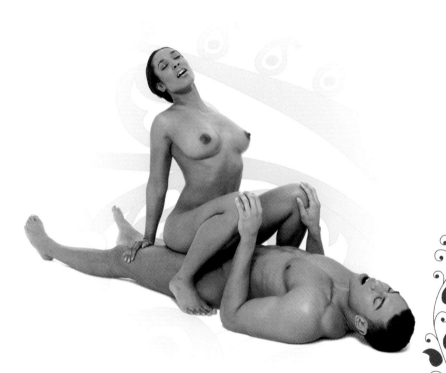

She sits on him, and leans back to support herself on his knees.

Divine moment: Make him submit to you.
Pure nirvana: "Listen to the sighs and heavy breathing of the woman.
They witness the violence of the bliss you have given her."

251 Blossom on the hillside

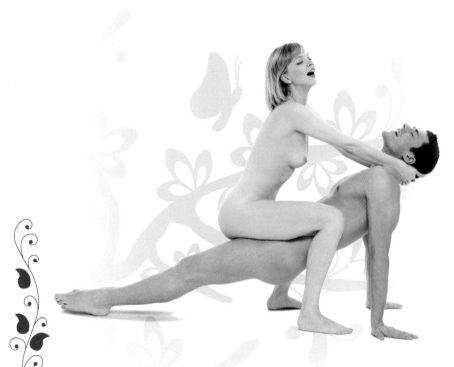

He makes an upward-facing ramp with his body, and she rides him.

Divine moment: Move into it from a flat-on-the-bed position.
Pure nirvana: Guys—try to keep everything rigid.

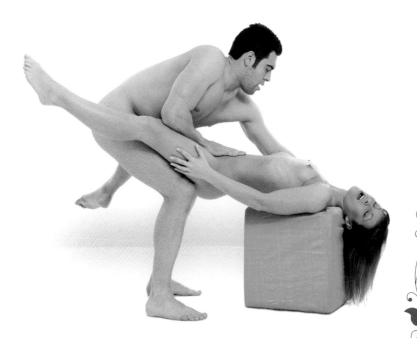

She lies on a raised surface, and he penetrates in a standing position.

Divine moment: You've just had dinner—you push the plates to one side and...
Pure nirvana: ...mmmmm, dessert.

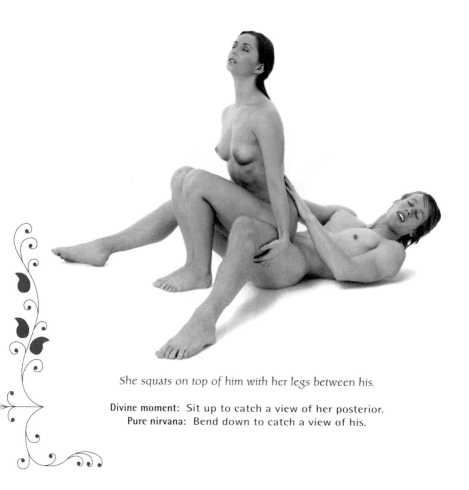

She squats on top of him with her legs between his.

Divine moment: Sit up to catch a view of her posterior.
Pure nirvana: Bend down to catch a view of his.

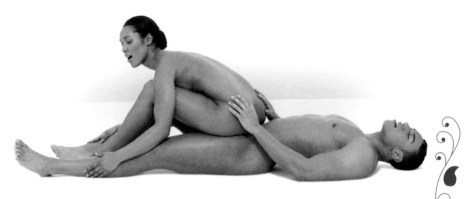

He lies flat then she sits on top, and leans toward his feet.

Divine moment: Run your fingers playfully over his lovesack.
Pure nirvana: Say hello to her perineum.

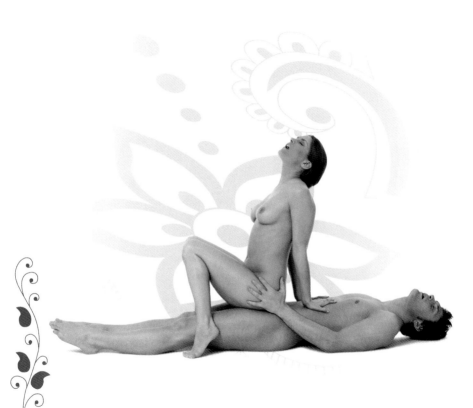

She sits on top with her hands on his torso.

Divine moment: Tell her it's time she sat down.
Pure nirvana: Guide her onto your waiting flute.

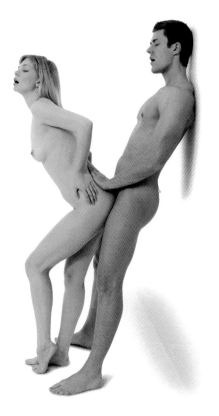

He leans against a wall, and she leans against him.

Divine moment: Say, "Rub my back, would you?"
Pure nirvana: Wiggle your butt into his crotch.

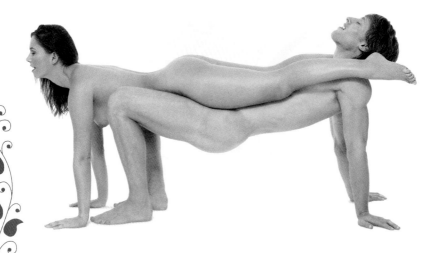

He makes his body into a table and she lies upon it with her hands on the floor.

Divine moment: "Bear her up like a bed."
Pure nirvana: Let the symmetry of your union mirror the
desires of your heart.

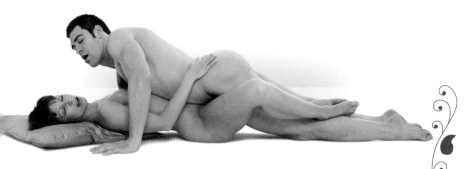

She positions her feet on the back of his knees as he penetrates from on top.

Divine moment: Draw his body close at the moment of supreme pleasure.
Pure nirvana: "If you wish to repeat the act, perfume yourself
with sweet odors."

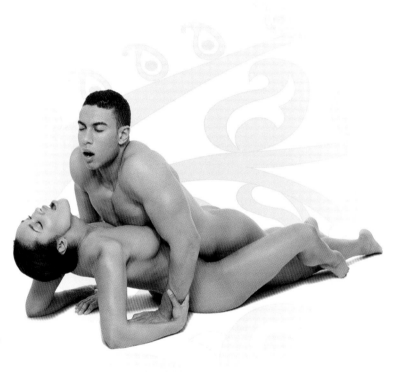

*He pulls himself up along the front of her body as she leans
back on her elbows.*

Divine moment: Guys—surf each wave of pleasure.
Pure nirvana: Prolong the inevitable moment by taking deep breaths.

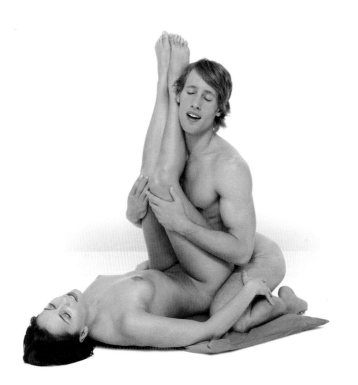

He pulls her legs close together, and hooks them over one shoulder.

Divine moment: Grip his member tightly.
Pure nirvana: Raise her off the bed, and push in deeper.

261 The toothpick

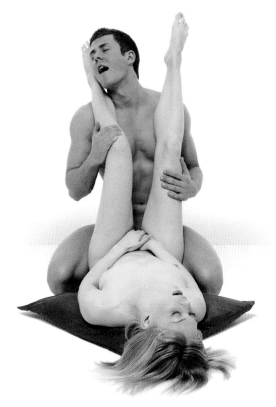

He sits on his heels, and holds her legs along the front of his body.

Divine moment: Guys—"introduce your member, and explore the
vagina from top to bottom and on all sides."
Pure nirvana: Girls—enjoy the movements of his "vigorous instrument."

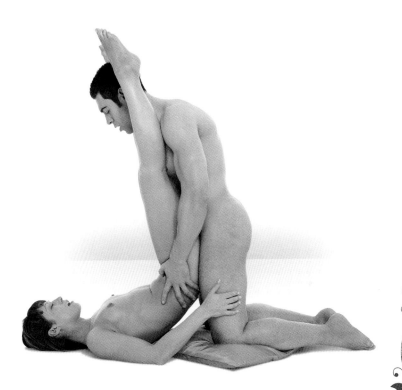

She aligns her ass with his pelvis, and points her legs to the ceiling.

Divine moment: Pause for a moment at the peak.
Pure nirvana: Gaze into each other's eyes.

263 The bold plunge

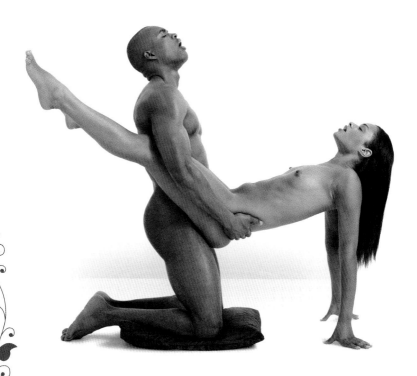

He pulls her onto him as he kneels, and she balances on her hands.

Divine moment: Link your hands beneath her back.
Pure nirvana: Or offer her a rapelling harness.

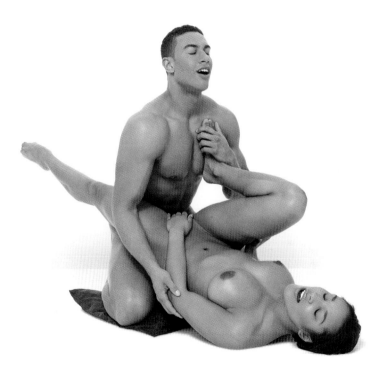

He kneels upright, and holds her off the ground with one foot flat on his chest and the other pointing behind him.

Divine moment: Penetrate a little way, then stop.
Pure nirvana: Then, in one fast stroke, enter completely.

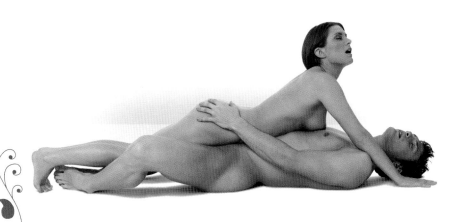

She lies on top of him with her head and shoulders raised.

Divine moment: Wait until his member is truly prominent
before you take it inside.
Pure nirvana: To kiss him, you "need only lay your arms on the bed."

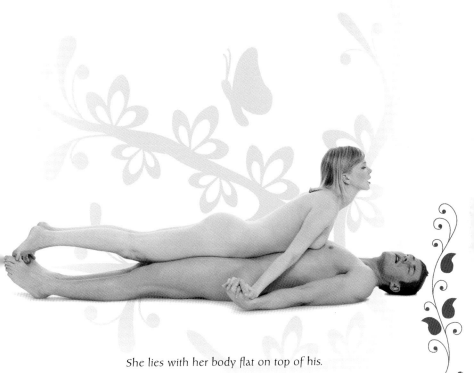

She lies with her body flat on top of his.

Divine moment: Oil your fronts first.
Pure nirvana: Slide your way to the heavenly palace of bliss.

267 Belly press

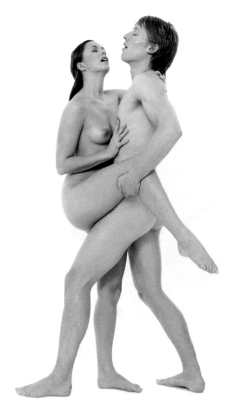

They stand facing each other, and he lifts her thigh in his hand.

Divine moment: Do it during a sudden moment of lust.
Pure nirvana: Gasp an urgent "I want you."

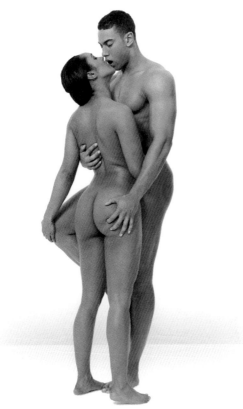

He faces her in a standing position with one foot pressed against his calf.

Divine moment: Reveal your intentions by pressing your bamboo rod against her navel.
Pure nirvana: Respond by kissing him.

269 Two bamboo stems

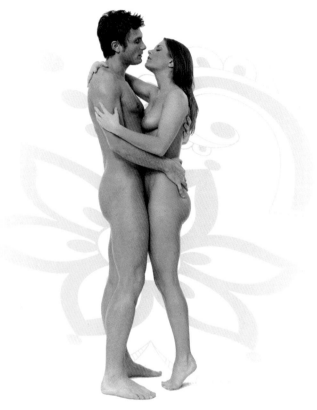

They stand with their bodies pressed together so they can feel each other's breath.

Divine moment: Feel the sexual tension mount.
Pure nirvana: Reach down to handle his lingam.

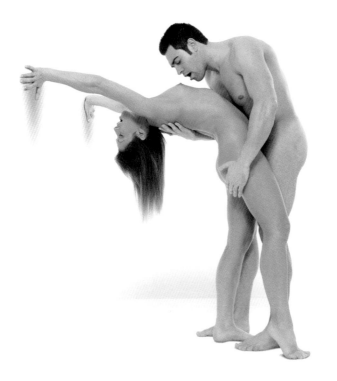

She does a half backbend against the nearest wall.

Divine moment: Can't penetrate her lower deck? Kiss her upper deck instead.
Pure nirvana: Trust him to catch you.

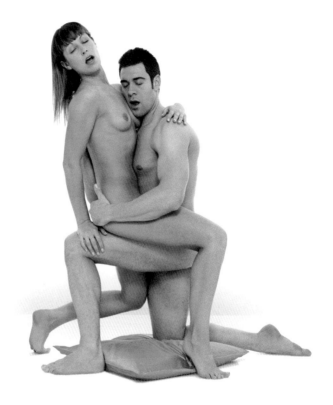

They face each other in a half-kneeling position.

Divine moment: Work together to get jiggy.
Pure nirvana: cross another tricky maneuver off the list.

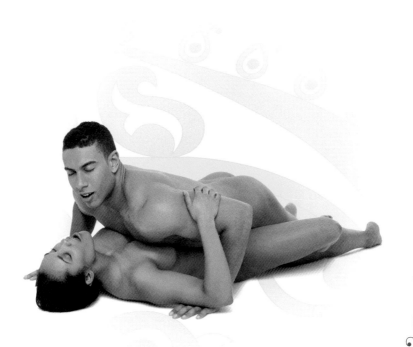

He gets on top, and she puts her feet on the back of his legs.

Divine moment: Make it sheet-ripping and mattress-pounding.
Pure nirvana: Guys—take an oral sex break if you need to slow down.

The worshiper

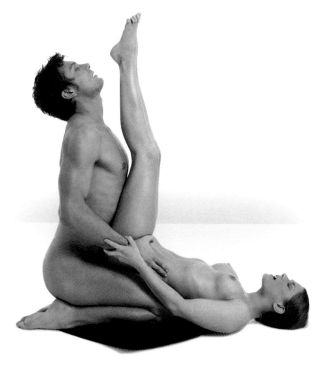

She rests her bum on his thighs, and points her toes skyward.

Divine moment: Go the kinky route—tie her ankles together.
Pure nirvana: Use soft leg cuffs.

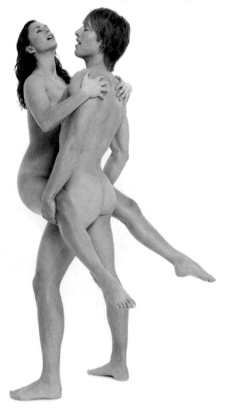

He picks her up, and pulls her onto him.

Divine moment: Do it when his peg is ready to pop.
Pure nirvana: Make your thrusts small but efficient.

275 The easy posture

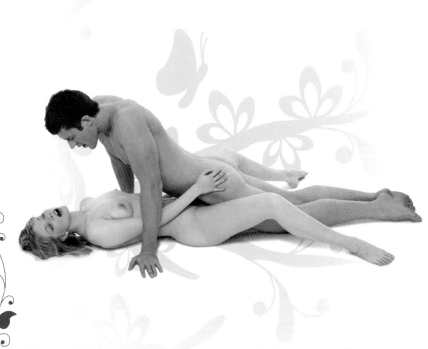

She opens her legs and, keeping his arms straight, he penetrates from on top.

Divine moment: Do it late at night to help you sleep.
Pure nirvana: Try it instead of hot milk.

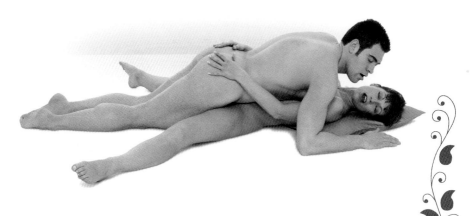

She lies on her back, and parts her legs wide to let him in.

Divine moment: Do it with a new beau.
Pure nirvana: Try each other on for fit.

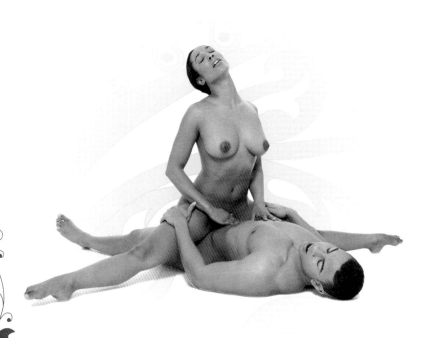

He lies back while she does the splits on top of him.

Divine moment: Girls—dress for the occasion.
Pure nirvana: A feather boa and heels.

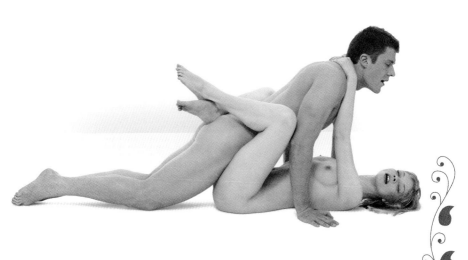

He does a kneeling push-up, and she winds her arms and legs around him.

Divine moment: Make it warm, intimate, and romantic.
Pure nirvana: Stay wrapped in your cocoon afterward.

279 The cricket

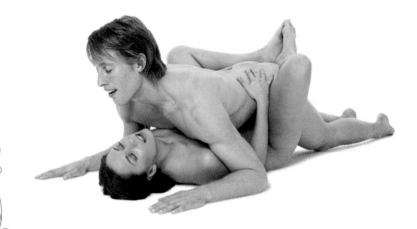

He lies on top of her, and she presses the soles of her feet together behind him.

Divine moment: Move in a way you know she likes.
Pure nirvana: Join lips and tongues.

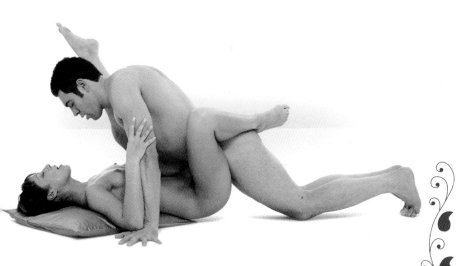

She lies beneath him with one leg around his waist, and one over his shoulder.

Divine moment: Get hot, sweaty, and breathless.
Pure nirvana: Steam up the windows.

281 Two fish

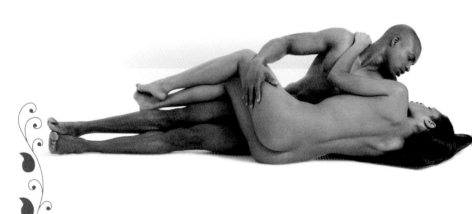

They lie facing on their sides. She drapes her legs over him so that her feet rest on his calves.

Divine moment: Undulate gently.
Pure nirvana: To get him in, twist so your fish are flush.

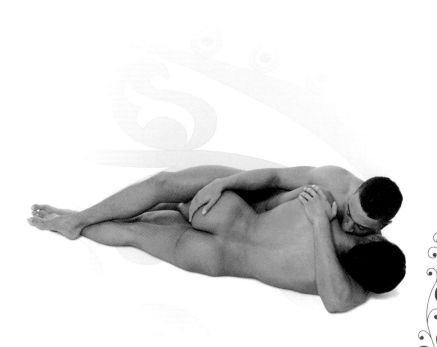

He folds his upper leg over hers as they lie facing on their sides.

Divine moment: Guys—do your best seduction moves.
Pure nirvana: Softly kiss the side of her neck.

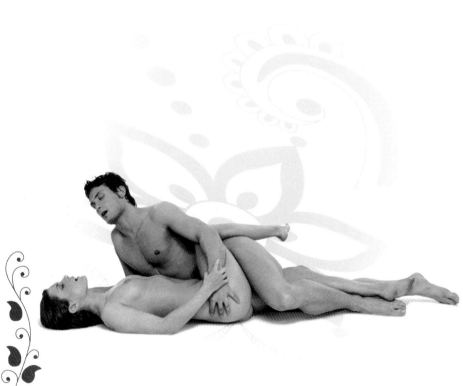

She lies in a semi-twist with her leg over his waist. He lies on his side.

Divine moment: Take a leisurely approach.
Pure nirvana: Untwine and re-entwine.

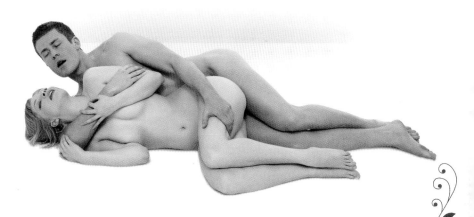

He makes a rear entry as she lies on her side with her knees drawn up.

Divine moment: Use it as a nonverbal goodnight.
Pure nirvana: Stay joined as you drift off to sleep.

285 Huge bird above a dark sea

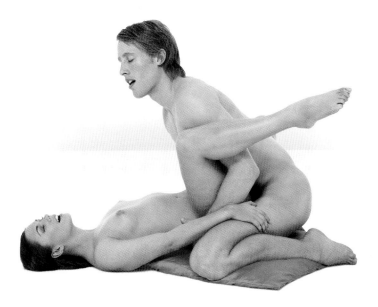

He kneels before her, and she opens up her legs to clasp him.

Divine moment: Twirl your huge bird on her love button before you enter.
Pure nirvana: Pull out, and repeat at regular intervals.

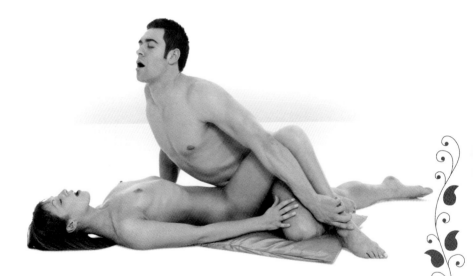

He reaches back and grasps her right ankle, while supporting himself with his right arm.

Divine moment: Swoop down on her like a bird sighting its prey.
Pure nirvana: Arch your backs to achieve the perfect union of opposites.

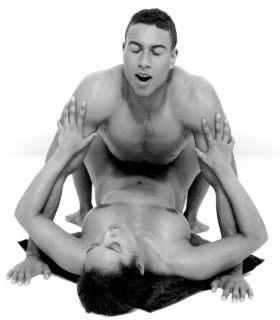

He is raised above her in a push-up position, and she brings her hips to meet him.

Divine moment: Get into a body-slamming rhythm.
Pure nirvana: Let lightning bolts rip through you.

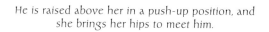

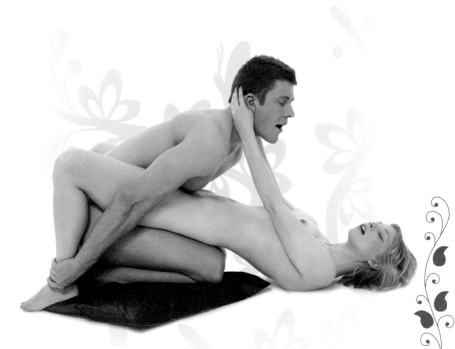

*He grips her ankles as she rests her hips on his lap
and her shoulders on the bed.*

Divine moment: Guys—lean forward like a jockey on a speeding horse.
Pure nirvana: Concentrate on passing the finish line together.

289 The dragonfly

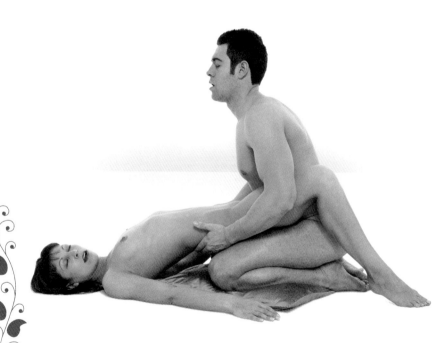

He kneels on his heels and supports her in a lying position on his lap.

Divine moment: Give her a three-handed massage (two hands plus member).
Pure nirvana: Synchronize the movements of all three "hands."

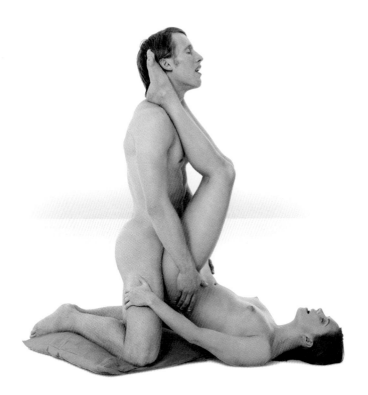

He kneels upright, and she rests her feet on his shoulders.

Divine moment: Stretch your legs so they're "tall like a pine tree."
Pure nirvana: But keep them flexible—like a pine tree in the wind.

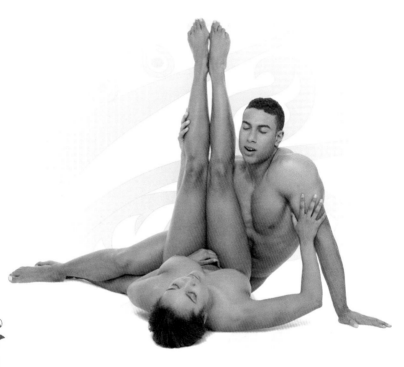

She raises her legs in a straight line, and he lies perpendicular to her.

Divine moment: Nuzzle the back of her knees.
Pure nirvana: Graze his arms with your fingernails.

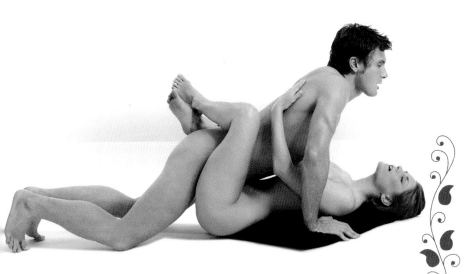

He supports himself on his hands and knees, and she wraps
her limbs around him.

Divine moment: Lie over her like a pine tree falling to the ground.
Pure nirvana: Girls—pull him close to your body.

293 Path through a narrow gorge

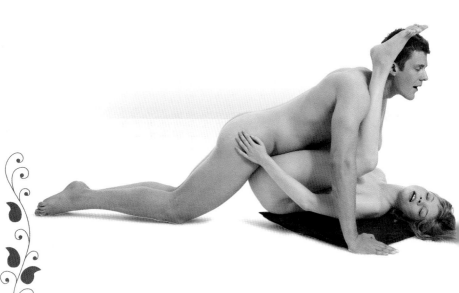

From the missionary position, she moves her feet over his shoulders.

Divine moment: Move with exquisite slowness.
Pure nirvana: Lock your arms so she feels the weight of your member
but not your body.

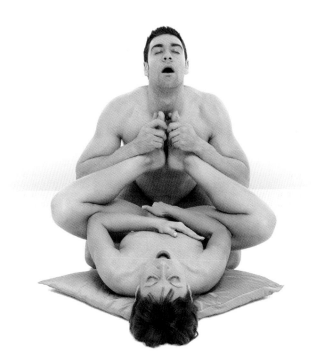

He grabs her feet, and presses her soles together as she lies on the floor.

Divine moment: Girls—do it as a groin-stretching exercise.
Pure nirvana: Compliment her on her supple body.

295 Phoenix playing in a red cave

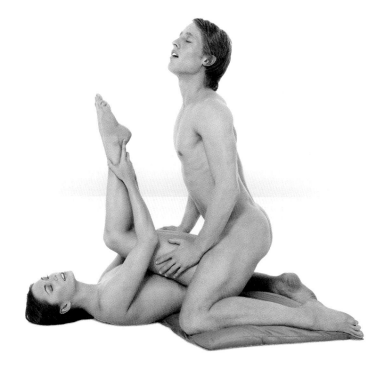

He enters in a kneeling position as she lies back clasping her ankles.

Divine moment: Guys—enter and withdraw from her 72 times.
Pure nirvana: Girls—feel the flow of chi to your red cave.

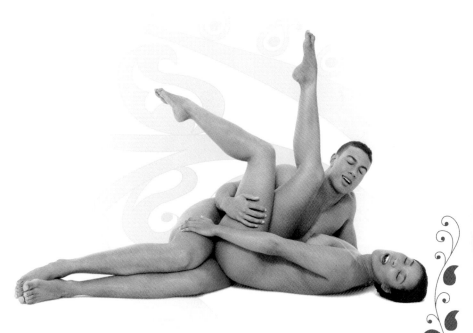

He makes a side entry as she lies on her back.

Divine moment: Savor the new angle of penetration.
Pure nirvana: Discover hotspots you didn't know existed.

297 Horse pulling a cart

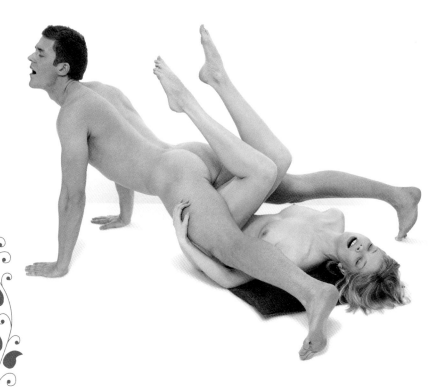

He gets into a push-up position, and she lies with her head between his feet
and her legs raised over his ass.

Divine moment: Show off your amazing backward-bending member.
Pure nirvana: Treat it as penis yoga.

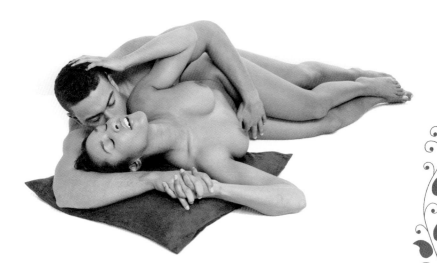

They lie on their sides with him behind; she twists to caress him.

Divine moment: Do it on your wedding night.
Pure nirvana: Mandarin ducks symbolize a happy, faithful marriage.

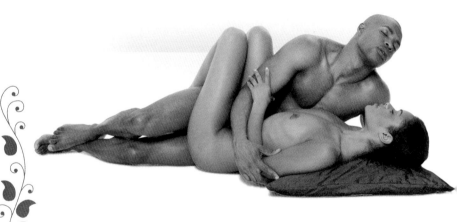

He lies on his side, and she lies on her back with her legs over his waist.

Divine moment: Enjoy the face-to-face intimacy...
Pure nirvana: ...plus deep penetration.

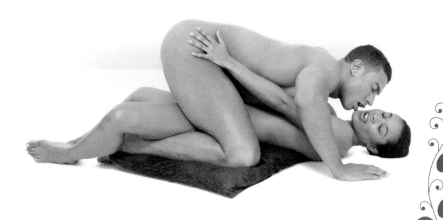

He lies on top of her with his knees on either side of her waist.

Divine moment: Make it hot, messy, and sweaty.
Pure nirvana: Use your nails on him.

301 Crouching tiger

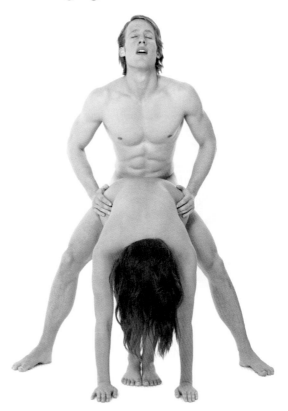

She crouches with her hands on the floor, and he takes her from behind.

Divine moment: Do it when you get home drunk.
Pure nirvana: Stumble into bed for the second act.

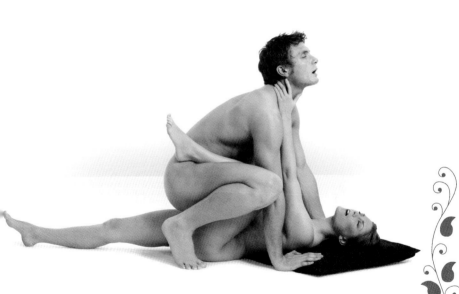

He squats over her, and she hooks one ankle over his hip.

Divine moment: Hold his head in your hands.
Pure nirvana: Put your fingers in his mouth.

303 Seagulls on the wing

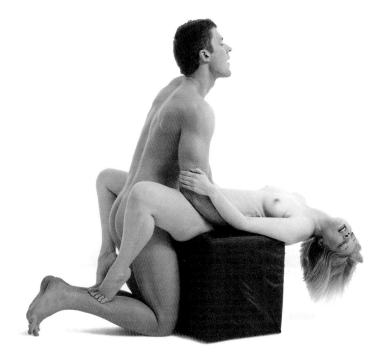

She lies back on a low surface, and he kneels between her legs.

Divine moment: Guys—begin with some moan-creating cunnilingus.
Pure nirvana: Follow with a swift, piercing insertion.

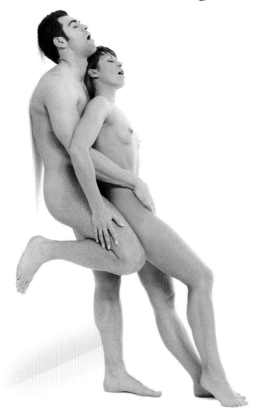

She presses her back against his belly as he leans with one foot against a wall.

Divine moment: Do it after feverish standing-up sex.
Pure nirvana: Make it your orgasm come-down position.

305 Flower among bamboo

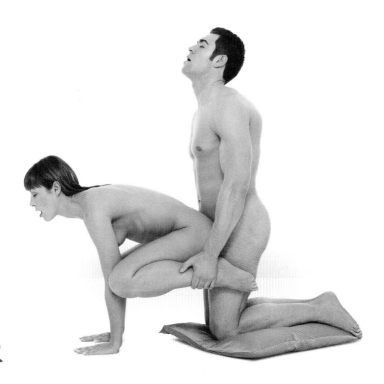

He kneels upright and lifts her onto him with her legs bent and her hands on the floor.

Divine moment: Press yourself between her cheeks.
Pure nirvana: Cover yourself in lube to ensure a smooth passage.

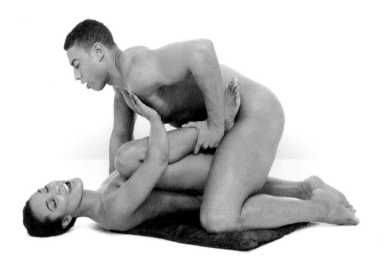

He gets on top, and she plants her heel in his groin and her hand on his chest.

Divine moment: Try to push him off.
Pure nirvana: Play the "no, you-can't-have-me" game.

307 The dragon turns

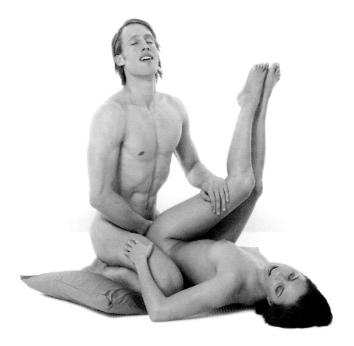

She raises her legs, and he kneels with his thighs around her hips.

Divine moment: He churns his dragon's head on her love bean.
Pure nirvana: Don't stop until she explodes.

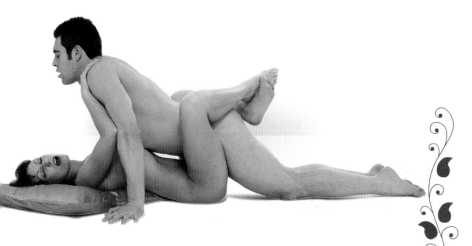

She lies on her back with him on top; she crosses her feet behind his bum.

Divine moment: Guys—stop when you're approaching the gate.
Pure nirvana: Cool down then start all over again.

309 Butterflies in flight

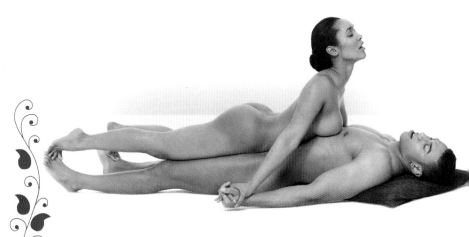

He lies flat on his back, and she aligns her body on top.

Divine moment: Brace yourself against his hands and feet.
Pure nirvana: Rub your pearl against his pubic bone.

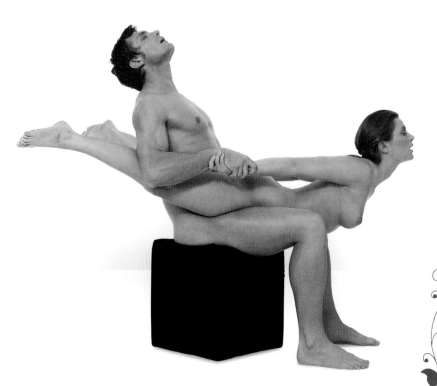

He sits on a stool or block, and she gets into a flying position with her thighs around his torso.

Divine moment: Slide your fish into her pond.
Pure nirvana: Try the weightless option—do it in a swimming pool.

311 Butterfly

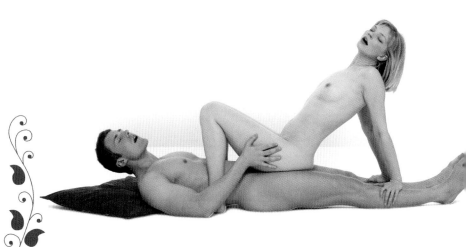

She sits astride his prone body with her hands resting on his calves.

Divine moment: Girls—do what you want with him.
Pure nirvana: Guys—address her as ma'am.

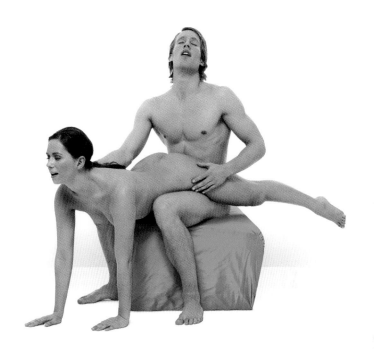

He sits, and she puts her hands on the floor and clasps his waist with her thighs.

Divine moment: Start by sliding sexily onto his lap.
Pure nirvana: Then walk your hands forward until they're on the floor.

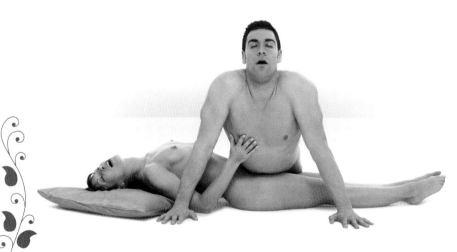

313 Plucking an instrument

She lies on her back, and he lies at right angles across her middle.

Divine moment: Find bliss if you own a side-bending shaft.
Pure nirvana: Or just thrust between her oiled thighs.

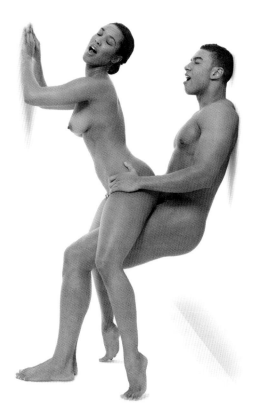

He gets into a semi-sitting position, and she straddles him.

Divine moment: Brace yourself against a wall on either side.
Pure nirvana: Do it in corridors, hallways, alleyways, back passages....

315 Cat and mouse sharing a hole

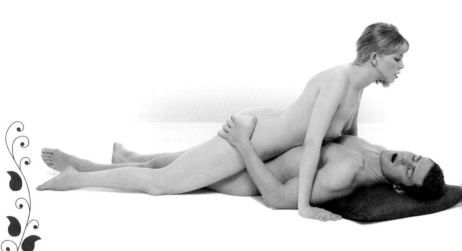

She lies on top of his body with her legs on either side of his.

Divine moment: Keep rolling over so you alternate being on top.
Pure nirvana: Pretend you're "a cat and mouse fighting for a hole."

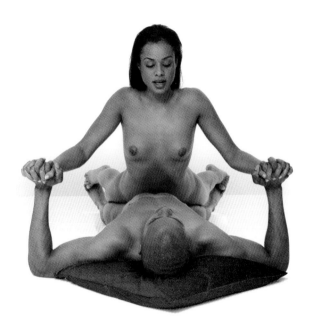

She lies on top of him and, supporting herself on his hands,
raises her head and chest.

Divine moment: Make your bodies long and taut.
Pure nirvana: Feel a delicious stretch in your genitals.

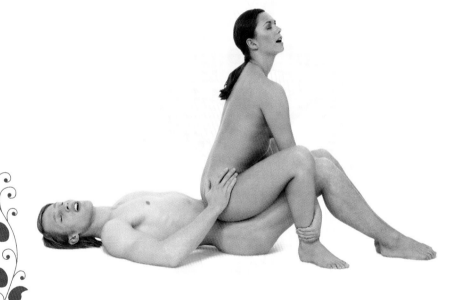

She squats on top of him facing his feet.

Divine moment: Make it his birthday treat...
Pure nirvana: ...after the lap dance, and the blow job.

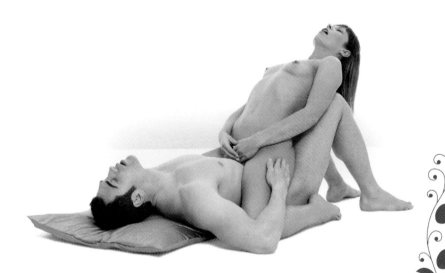

He lies with his knees bent, and she lies back on his thighs.

Divine moment: Girls—hold a vibrator against your lily pad.
Pure nirvana: Turn it up to max speed.

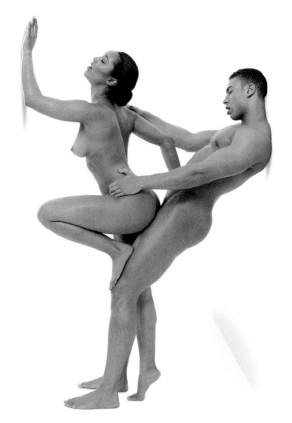

He stands behind, and penetrates her as she presses one foot against his thigh.

Divine moment: Do it after your parents have visited.
Pure nirvana: Wave goodbye through the window.

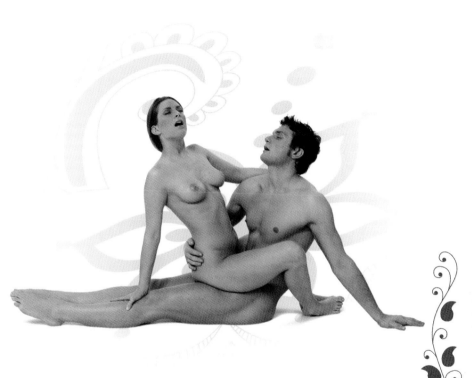

He sits with his legs straight, and she lowers herself onto him in a semi-twist.

Divine moment: Play some rousing opera.
Pure nirvana: Synchronize your climax with the crescendo.

321 Falling petals

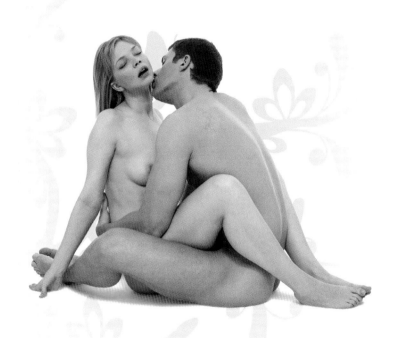

They sit face to face with their feet behind each other's back.

Divine moment: Do it after a candlelit bath.
Pure nirvana: Inhale the scent of each other.

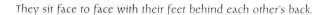

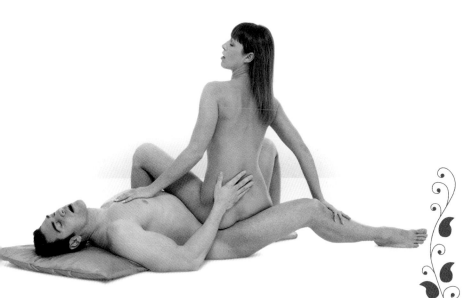

He lies on his back with his knees apart—she takes a seat.

Divine moment: Ride him side saddle.
Pure nirvana: Lean back on your hands, and thrust your hips.

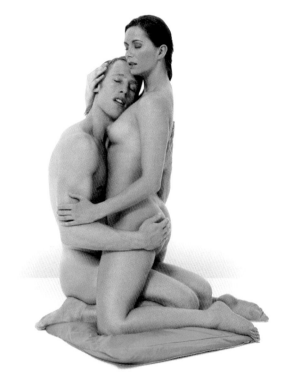

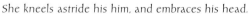

She kneels astride his him, and embraces his head.

Divine moment: Do it when he wants a bosom for a pillow.
Pure nirvana: Girls—think maternal yet sexy.

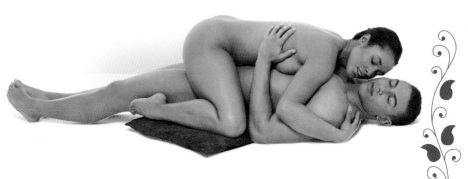

She lies on top, and cuddles him with her knees drawn up.

Divine moment: Do it when you're in the mood for sweet lovin'.
Pure nirvana: Stay in position for a cozy come-down.

325 Snake crossing a path

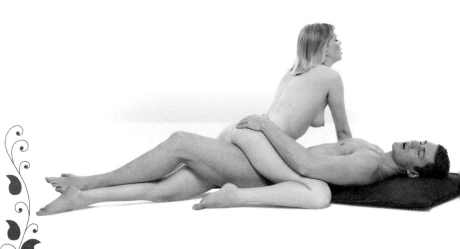

She lies diagonally across his body with one leg straight, and one leg bent.

Divine moment: Girls—"tighten your muscles, and agitate your hips."
Pure nirvana: "Agitate both to the left and the right."

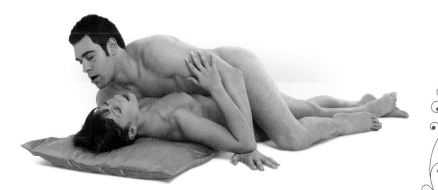

He's on top, and she's underneath with one leg between his.

Divine moment: Guys—press against one side of her cinnabar grotto and then the other.

Pure nirvana: Hang onto your juice for as long as you can.

327 Cicada on a bough

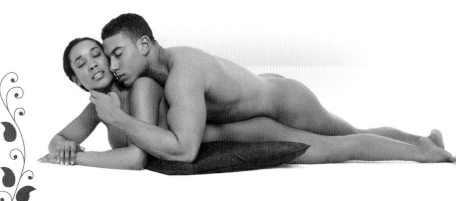

She lies on her tummy. He lies on top, his legs between hers.

Divine moment: Make up silly terms of endearment.
Pure nirvana: Whisper like cicadas at dusk.

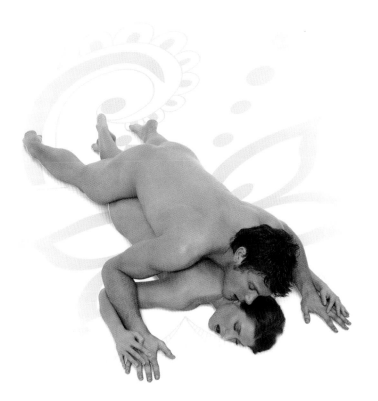

She lies flat on her tummy, and he covers her body with his.

Divine moment: Introduce your doodle to her rosebud.
Pure nirvana: Check before you charge in.

329 Bird of paradise

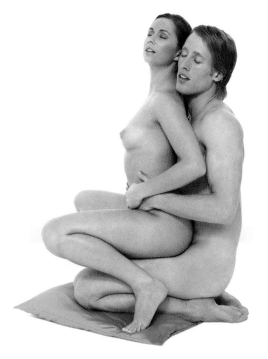

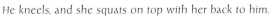

He kneels, and she squats on top with her back to him.

Divine moment: Do it in the bathtub...
Pure nirvana: ...with the aid of a vibrating rubber duck.

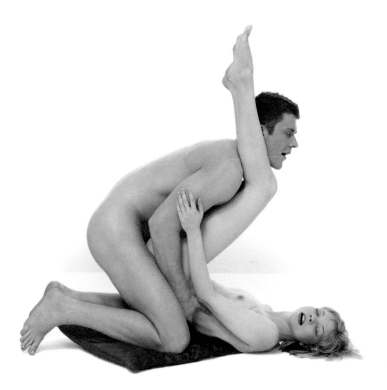

She raises her knees, and rests her calves on his shoulders as he enters.

Divine moment: Guys—you play the ape.
Pure nirvana: Girls—you play Jane.

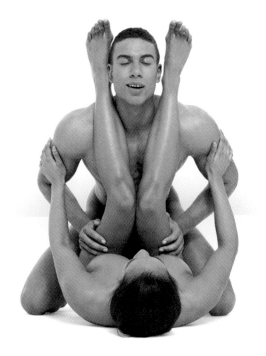

He holds her legs against his front, and leans over her body.

Divine moment: Give yourself up to toe-biting, skin-scratching intensity.
Pure nirvana: Gasp each other's name.

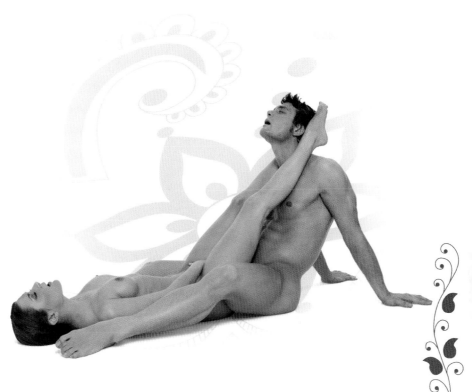

*He stretches out his legs alongside her body, she rests
her ankles on his shoulders.*

Divine moment: Make your body taut by stretching your arms over your head.
Pure nirvana: Feel the chi flowing into you.

333 The spring goat

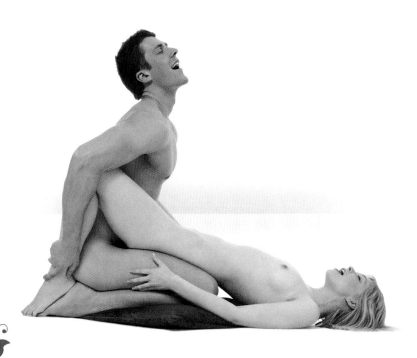

She presses her feet against his, and lies back over his lap.

Divine moment: Say, "Baby, I wanna touch your sole."
Pure nirvana: Use his feet as a push-off point.

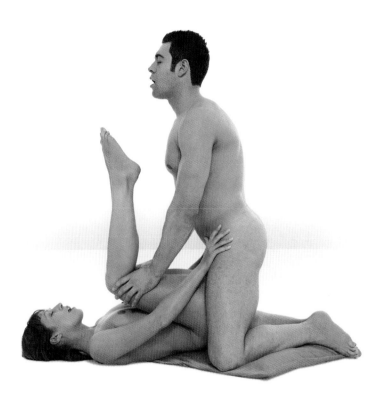

She brings her knees to her chest while he enters in an upright kneel.

Divine moment: Make your movements slow.
Pure nirvana: And your penis hard.

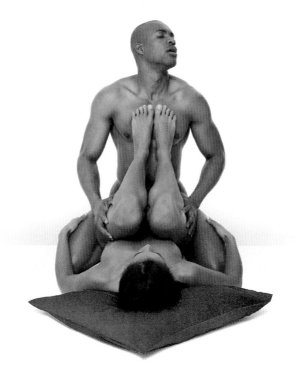

He puts his knees on either side of her hips, and she rests her feet on his chest.

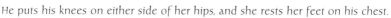

Divine moment: Apply foot pressure to make him thrust deeper or shallower.
Pure nirvana: Feel the crackle of sexual energy.

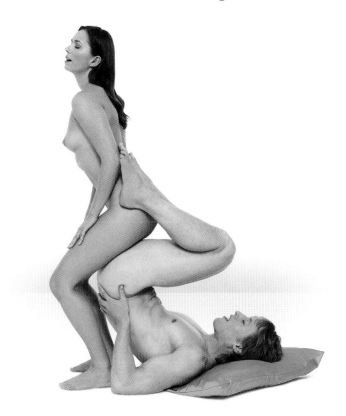

He does a half-shoulderstand, and she perches on his ass.

Divine moment: Guys—bend your penis, and slip her the tip.
Pure nirvana: Treat it as a taster session.

337 Horse shakes feet

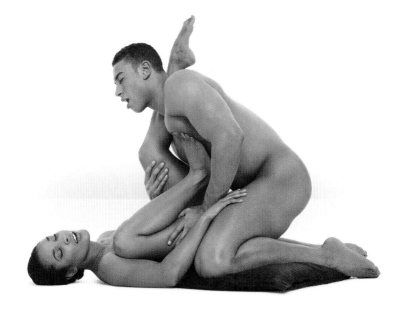

She puts one foot on his chest, and one over his shoulder.

Divine moment: Tweak his nipple with your toes.
Pure nirvana: Move like a piece of well-oiled machinery.

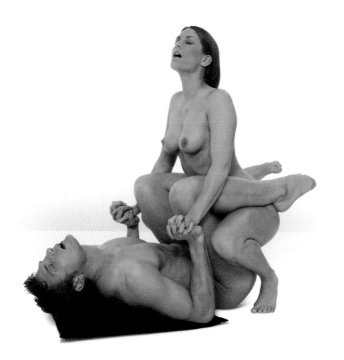

He brings his knees to his chest, and she lowers herself onto him.

Divine moment: Get a firm grip on his hands.
Pure nirvana: Girls—try it facing away.

339 The jade joint

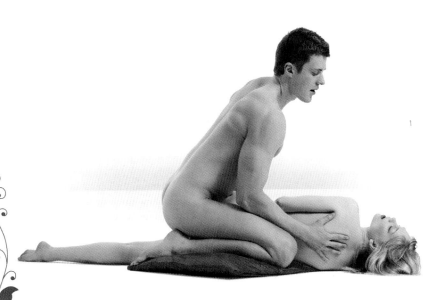

She lies on her side with one knee raised. He straddles and enters.

Divine moment: Press your fingertips into her back...
Pure nirvana: ...and your jade stalk into her jade gate.

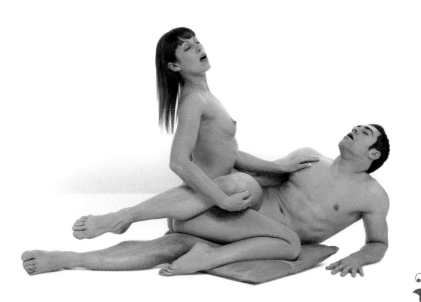

He turns on one side, and hooks one leg around the front of her waist.

Divine moment: Pleasure yourselves on each other's thigh.
Pure nirvana: Tease, but do not penetrate.

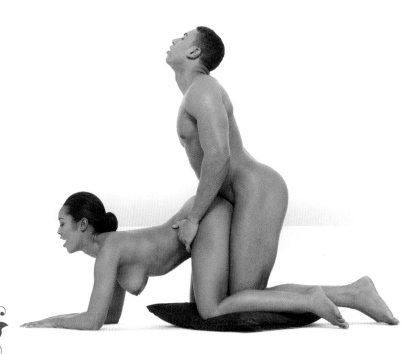

He takes her from behind as she rests on her knees and forearms.

Divine moment: Guys—growl with lust.
Pure nirvana: Girls—purr with passion.

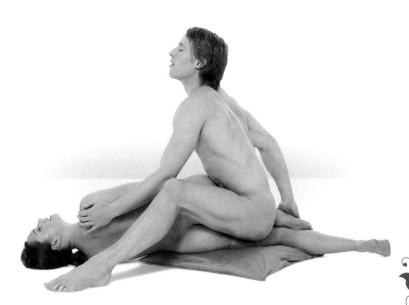

She lies on her side with one knee drawn up while he sits and straddles.

Divine moment: Insert your member by a few inches.
Pure nirvana: Tell him when he hits your G-spot.

343 Tiger step

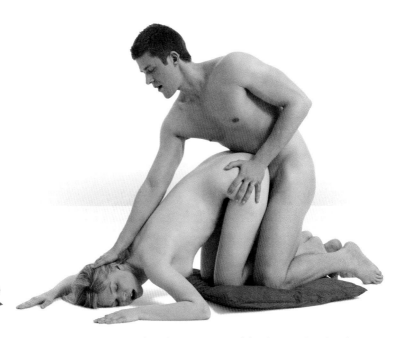

*He penetrates in a kneeling position while she puts her head
on the floor and her butt in the air.*

Divine moment: Put one hand on her butt, and one on her head.
Pure nirvana: Make it part of a sub/dom roleplay.

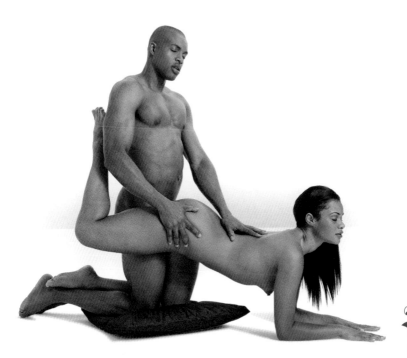

He takes her doggie style as she cocks a leg in the air.

Divine moment: Guys—virtually withdraw on each stroke.
Pure nirvana: Plunge deeply when you feel the rain coming.

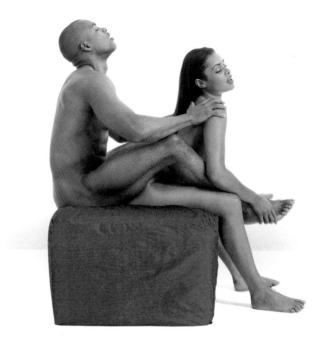

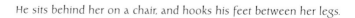

He sits behind her on a chair, and hooks his feet between her legs.

Divine moment: Massage her shoulders with your hands...
Pure nirvana: ...and her thighs with your feet.

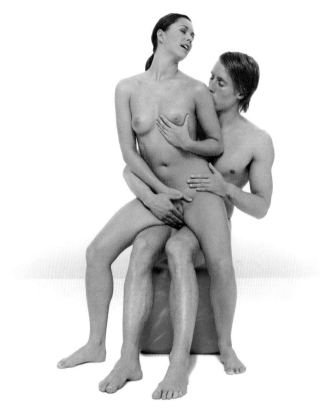

He's in a chair, and she takes a seat on his lap.

Divine moment: Bend over in front of him then sink slowly onto his member.
Pure nirvana: Guys—"scratch yourself like a goat on a tree."

347 Late spring donkey

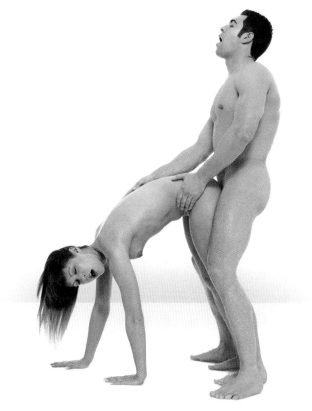

She puts her hands on the floor, and he takes her squarely from behind.

Divine moment: Do it when you're so hot you can't wait.
Pure nirvana: Lift her dress, and drop your trousers.

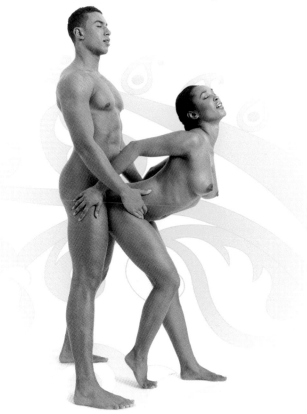

She curves her ass into his body in a semi-standing position.

Divine moment: Do it in a toilet stall.
Pure nirvana: Bite your lip, and try not to make a sound.

349 Two trees

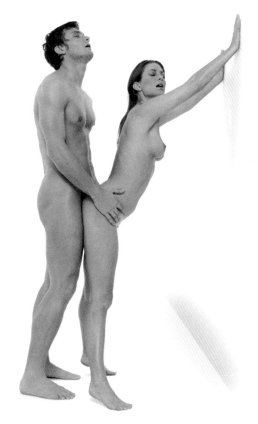

She has her palms flat against a wall, and he stands behind her.

Divine moment: Offer to help her hang the wallpaper.
Pure nirvana: Get sticky together.

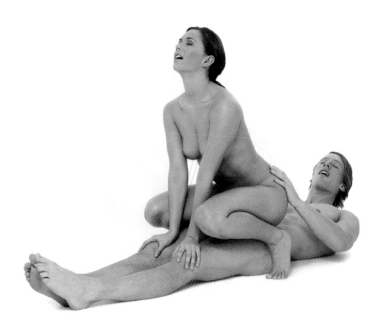

She squats on top of him with her hands on his knees.

Divine moment: Guys—make long hand-over-hand strokes on her back.
Pure nirvana: Girls—bob up and down like a rabbit.

351 Rabbit on the ground

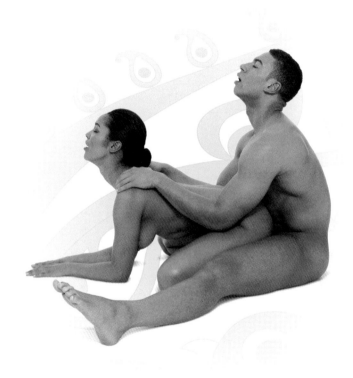

She kneels with her legs widely opened, and her breasts close to the ground.

Divine moment: Do it alfresco on top of a picnic blanket.
Pure nirvana: Take a post-coital nap under the blanket.

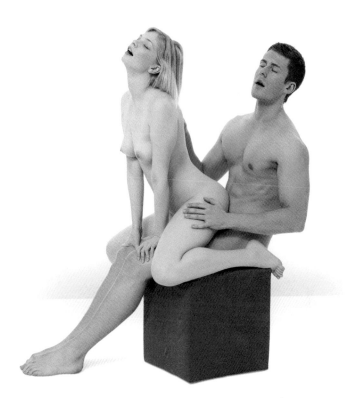

She kneels astride him as he sits in a chair.

Divine moment: Do it on the couch during a commercial break.
Pure nirvana: Close your eyes, mute the TV, and move fast.

353 The empress

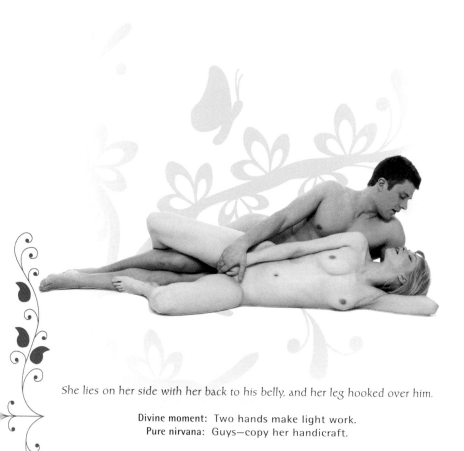

She lies on her side with her back to his belly, and her leg hooked over him.

Divine moment: Two hands make light work.
Pure nirvana: Guys—copy her handicraft.

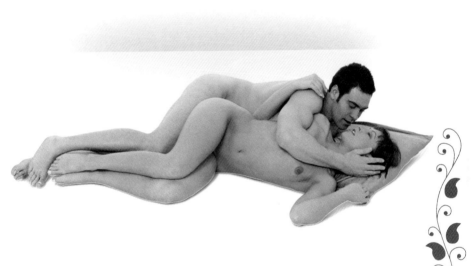

He lies behind her in a spoons position, and caresses her face.

Divine moment: Relax into low-energy lovin'.
Pure nirvana: Make it your hangover cure.

355 Forest pines

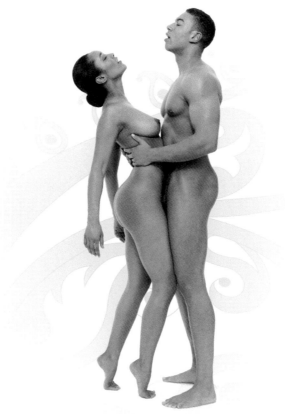

They stand face to face, and press against each other.

Divine moment: Thrust at full throttle between her thighs.
Pure nirvana: Girls—height incompatibility? Stand on a step.

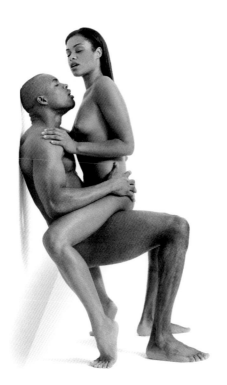

He leans against a wall to make a chair with his body. She sits astride him.

Divine moment: Slide appreciatively onto his strong thighs.
Pure nirvana: Take the relaxing route—do it on a real chair.

357 Autumn dog

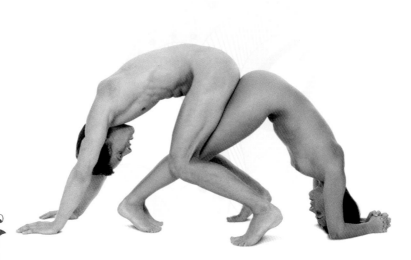

They press their buttocks together as they make intersecting arches.

Divine moment: Push your ass high in the air, "like a dog in heat."
Pure nirvana: Nod and wink while you're down there.

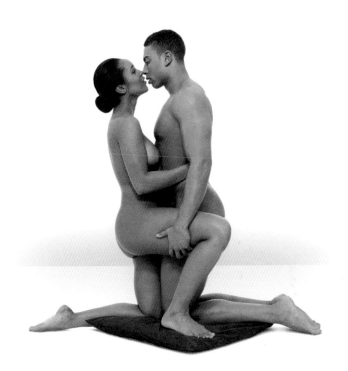

They kneel with their bodies pressed together; she has one foot flat on the ground.

Divine moment: Guys—take your shaft firmly in your hand...
Pure nirvana: ...and move its tip against her tip.

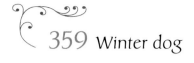

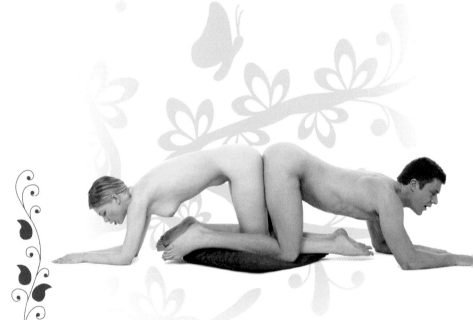

They both rest on knees and forearms with their butts pushed together.

Divine moment: Wag your tails.
Pure nirvana: Get off on butt frottage.

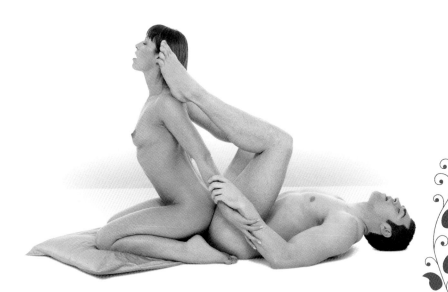

He lies back with his feet propped on her shoulders.

Divine moment: Bend his penis in a new direction (*slowly*).
Pure nirvana: Or—easier—get connected with a double-ended dildo.

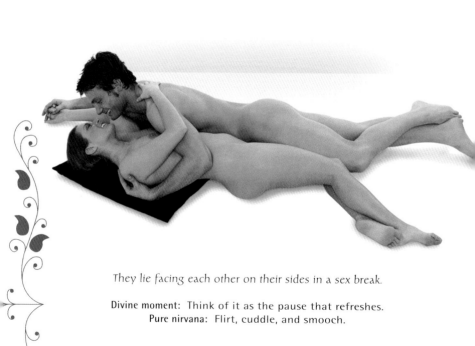

They lie facing each other on their sides in a sex break.

Divine moment: Think of it as the pause that refreshes.
Pure nirvana: Flirt, cuddle, and smooch.

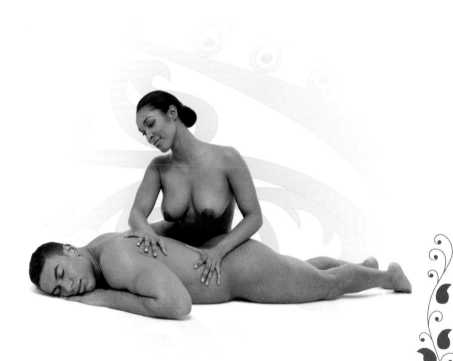

He lies on his belly while she massages his back.

Divine moment: Smooth your palms over him as though planing a piece of wood.
Pure nirvana: Guys—drift off to another dimension.

363 Evening rain

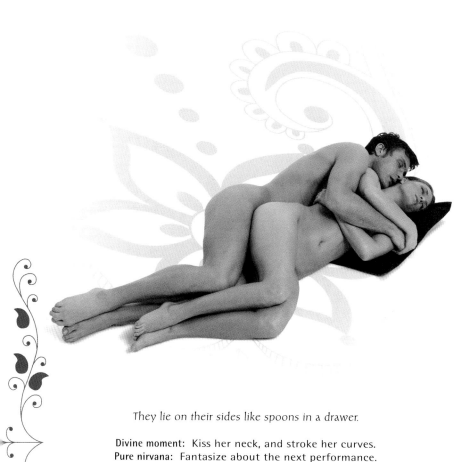

They lie on their sides like spoons in a drawer.

Divine moment: Kiss her neck, and stroke her curves.
Pure nirvana: Fantasize about the next performance.

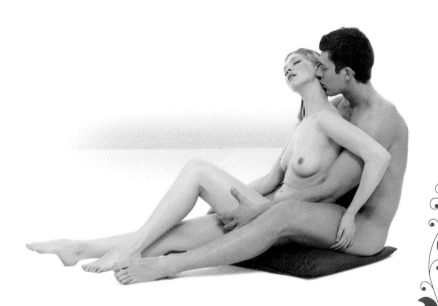

She sits in front of him enclosed by his legs.

Divine moment: Bask in post-sex euphoria.
Pure nirvana: Snuggle, snog, caress, canoodle.

365 Cicadas at night

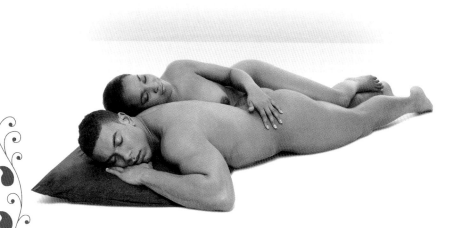

He lies on his belly while she cuddles him from the side.

Divine moment: Congratulate yourselves on an erotic marathon.
Pure nirvana: Take a well-earned snooze.

*Now it's time to start
all over again…*

Perfect positions for... sweet romance

You've been apart/you know it's love/you just got engaged

Perfect positions for... mind-blowing novelty

You're out to impress/you want a workout/you're bored with missionary

Perfect positions for... steaming up the windows with lust

You're mad with desire/it's been ages/you've been propositioned

Perfect positions for... the erotic quickie

The boss is out/your parents are due/it's almost time to pick up the kids

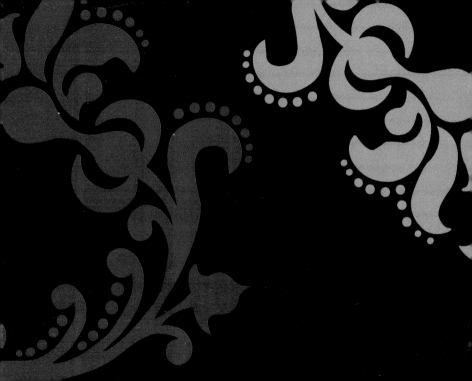